Ayahuasca

Exploration of Consciousness
Through Plant Medicine

*(A Comprehensive Guide to Understanding
Ayahuasca and It's Healing Power)*

Bernard Boyd

Published By **Darby Connor**

Bernard Boyd

Ayahuasca: Exploration of Consciousness Through Plant Medicine (A Comprehensive Guide to Understanding Ayahuasca and It's Healing Power)

ISBN   978-1-998038-43-5

Legal & Disclaimer

The information contained in this book is not designed to replace or take the place of any form of medicine or professional medical advice. The information in this book has been provided for educational & entertainment purposes only.

The information contained in this book has been compiled from sources deemed reliable, and it is accurate to the best of the Author's knowledge; however, the Author cannot guarantee its accuracy and validity and cannot be held liable for any errors or omissions. Changes are periodically made to this book. You must consult your doctor or get professional medical advice before using any of the suggested remedies, techniques, or information in this book.

Table Of Contents

Chapter 1: Nature's Gift

"Nature is the teacher of man. Her riches are open for him to explore, opens the eye, illuminates the mind and cleanses the heart. Her effect is emanated from the sights and sounds that are her life."

-Alfred Bernhard Nobel

Nature is full of mysterious - and you could even call it incredible ways to teach humans about all the things that are waiting for discovery. While thousands of natural resources were already found by us but there's plenty more to discover that we are yet to set our eyes.

With a one blow of wind or the bloom of a flower or a flash of lightning, we humans discover that nature is not just there as an aesthetic power on the earth and is not solely to ensure the survival of both animals and humans nature can be a way to teach humans about the existence of their species and its potential to grow humankind more.

Ayahuasca is among the mysteries of nature and in the same way an amazing gift from nature. It was first discovered in the past and is found throughout nature to this day. Strangely enough, there's no precise explanation for what exactly happened when Ayahuasca first came to be discovered. There are some who claim it was accidental, however other experts assert that it was discovered after thorough examination of various herbs. However, no matter the way Ayahuasca was found however, it's a fact that it's a gift of nature to the human race.

Chapter 2: What Is Ayahuasca?

Ayahuasca is a potent brew made from hallucinogenic (hallucination-inducing) plants. It is mostly employed as a form of medicine and a way to enter the realm of spirituality and mind. Ayahuasca consumption typically requires a guided ceremony led by a skilled shaman however, you can also drink the drink on your own.

Ayahuasca is well-known to a variety of different cultures, such as those of India, Columbia, Brazil, Peru, and Ecuador. Since it is a widely used product It is thought that there will have around 40 different names for Ayahuasca in the world. The most well-known terms for it include the words yage, Natema, Caapi and migi. In the language spoken in Shipibo it's called "oni", which means "cooked." They also refer to it as "oni kobin", which is "cooked with knowledge."

Additionally, the word "Ayahuasca" has a literal significance in one of the most popular languages spoken in South America: the

Quechua. The Quechua language is characterized by Ayahuasca is broken down into two words "aya" and "huasca." "Aya" means "soul" or "spirit", while "huasca" refers to "vine." The literal significance of the word in Quechua can be described as "vine of the spirit" and "vine of the soul." There are some traditions who refer to it as "La Purga", which refers to its therapeutic value, refers to cleansing or removing illnesses of the soul body, mind and the spirit.

Ayahuasca is a potent mixture believed to be a spiritual and physical healer. For those who believe in the practice, Ayahuasca is said to be among the most powerful natural gifts, since it's more than just an ordinary remedy and is regarded as to be a sacred medicine. It's a source of natural entheogens, which are believed to possess therapeutic and oracular benefits.

Ayahuasca is a beverage that is made of a mixture with Ayahuasca vine, which is also called the Banisteriopsis caapi, along with different herbal infusions. The Ayahuasca vine is a source of harmala alkaloids which are classified as monoamineoxidase inhibitors (MAOIs).

Ayahuasca can be mixed with plants that contain DMT. The most common plants used with the Banisteriopsis caapi are the leaves of the chacruna plant (Psychotria viridis), leaves of Diplopterys cabrerana (chagropanga/chaliponga), plants from Solanaceous genera, and leaves from the Brugmansia species (toe), and Brunfelsia species. Others DMT plants used include:

Psychotria carthagensis (amyruca)

Mimosa tenuiflora/M. hostiles (mimosa, jurema)

Desmanthus illinoensis (Illinois bundle weed)

Justicia pectoralis (tilo, chapantye)

Phalaris arundinacea (reed canary grass)

Phalaris aquaa/Phalaris tubrose (bulbous canary grass)

Acacia species (wattle)

Virola species (parika, epena)

Piptadenia peregrine/ Anadenanthera peregrina (cohoba, curuba yopo, zumaque)

MAOI plants which could be used to be able to replace B. Caapi include some of the following:

Peganum harmala (Syrian rue, aspand, esphand, harmal)

Passionflower (passiflora incarnata)

Cocoa (theobroma cacao)

Certain additives could include one of the following:

Coca leaves (erythroxylum coca)

Tobacco (nicotania tabacum, n. rustica)

Peyote (lopophora williamsii)

San Pedro (trichocereus pachanoi, t. peruviani, echinopsis pachanoi, e. peruviana)

DMT (dimethlytryptamine) can be described as an hallucinogenic drug that you may be found in the body in small quantities. The substance DMT has a structural resemblance to melatonin as well as serotonin and serotonin, both monoamines. If DMT is able to bind to neuronal receptors of the brain it causes modifications in moods, thoughts processes, as well as states of alertness.

It is crucial to use DMT in conjunction with MAOI (monoamine inhibits oxidase) for it to work. The reason is that monoamine oxide that is released through the stomach lining is able to destroy monoamines and other chemicals. Therefore, MAOI, or a chemical that inhibits monoamine oxidase allows DMT to be protected and be absorbed by the bloodstream. This is however, the case only when it comes to DMT which is consumed orally. When inhaled or injected, DMT escapes the digestive process, and may work, even if the MAOI has not been consumed in conjunction with it.

"Ayahuasca" is the name that was originally used for Ayahuasca grapevine (B.caapi) that is blended with Chacruna and Chagropanga. In the end, any mix of MAOI and DMT and DMT, was referred to as Ayahuasca and. But, many consider the alternatives to be ayahuasca analogs/anahuasca but not actually Ayahuasca.

This mix of different ingredients makes up the mixture. Because of the many possible mixtures of Ayahuasca concoctions, there may have a myriad of effects. outcomes differ as the combinations differ. It is important to are aware of the tea's components and the intended effect before you drink the tea. Beware of mixing Ayahuasca along with other substances until you are sure of how you're acting. It is tempting to combine psychedelics like peyote, Psilocybin, and other in the drink however the results could turn overwhelming and possibly deadly.

There are different varieties of Ayahuasca that are based on the specific culture in which it is utilized. For Indians There are variants of thunder. To people from Peru there are white, yellow, red and black variations. For the inhabitants of Ecuador There are distinct categories for women and men. This is a perfect example of how Ayahuasca can be found in many different forms depending on where you're where you are around the globe. The species of plants utilized in the drink can depend on what's local to you.

As with similar to other medicines all the various mixtures of the Ayahuasca mixture are formulated to serve different functions. They are that are meant to heal the soul, others to treat physical ailments, others to help with psychological healing, etc. So, before drinking the Ayahuasca concoction, one should know the effects they want to experience in order to select decide on the Ayahuasca mix that will be most effective to achieve that goal.

Reasons People Consume Ayahuasca

Ayahausca is believed to be a potent treatment. It is not a common practice to drink ayahuasca in a recreational way solely. Consuming Ayahuasca may make it appear as if you're in a state of death, however if adhere to the guidelines and are located within a secure environment there isn't the least bit of danger. It is possible to experience uncomfortable feelings and frightening visions, however apart from that there are also the possibility of experiencing deep revelations, and experience a sense of happiness.

Ayahuasca produces an extraordinary mental state. It breaks up the stifling mental structures that define your experience and takes you into an alternate reality, in which everything is possible. If you've gotten used to the normal, you should be prepared to be deprived of that from your life. The idea of living in a totally new world can be both frightening as well as liberating, based upon how you view the situation.

The legend says that shamans and wizards have been using Ayahuasca over hundreds of years to communicate with spirits and forces. According to legend, people drink it to reach the realm of being capable of doing special tasks that include divining the future, connect with the spirits of nature, communicate with the dead, comprehend and cure illness, resolve problems, and many other things.

Apart from its supernatural properties Ayahuasca can also be helpful for treating mental disorders. Recent research has proven Ayahuasca provides fast and lasting anti-anxiety and antidepressant properties. In addition, numerous research on Ayahuasca has proven it can trigger positive changes in life and is safe for users.

Additionally, one can use Ayahuasca to simply experience some new sensations. You won't be disappointed as Ayahuasca is among the most powerful psychedelics available. Amazing images and sound await those who are determined enough to drink the drink, however everything could go to be wasted if that experience as entertainment, and not holy. If one intends to gain value from an Ayahuasca session, they could take home treasures which can sustain them for the rest of their lives.

Being A Psychonaut

Psychonauts use drugs and methods to investigate their personal as well as outer worlds, experiencing altered states of mind. Psychonauts do this due to a variety of motives. The reasons for this are like this:

In order to discover the mysteries of the mind

For them to confront the repressed thoughts of their beliefs, thoughts, fears and hopes

To better understand themselves

Finding a solution to the problem that they cannot overcome, despite having thought about it and striving to get it gone

Chapter 3: History

Like I said earlier, there's no clear evidence regarding the origins of Ayahuasca usage. According to those who study history and scientists, who research Ayahuasca and its use, that there is a good chance the first time it was used was by tribes from the Amazon.

The prehistoric record of its discovery can never be discovered; there is insufficient evidence to document what occurred during this time period that was prior to the 16th century on the fringes of Amazon. It is because of the historical fact that Spanish conquistadors first arrived in the Amazon around the time of the 16th century. And it was the conquistadors who made the first records of indigenous people in the Amazon.

There's been a lot of debate about what exactly Ayahuasca came to be discovered, how it was first discovered, and the person who discovered it first. There are legends about Peru that suggest that Ayahuasca originated from "plant teachers", but there are others from Brazil and Brazil who claim that it was a revelation made by the king Solomon. It is also believed to be a conviction among some that it was among the tribes that were indigenous to the Amazon which first utilized Ayahuasca.

There is no precise time when the first time it was used however there is some evidence which puts its first usage at around 5,000 years old. There are those who believe it was employed just about two thousand years ago because of the discovery of ceremonial vessels with trace amounts of Ayahuasca. However, the only thing to be certain about is Ayahuasca was first discovered years ago.

Although there's no specific evidence as to the first time it was used or the individuals that first used it, the most important thing is the fact that Ayahuasca was created and that people the present can benefit from it to enhance their personal lives.

Chapter 4: The Role Of Shamans

As Ayahuasca is a considered to be to be a sacred remedy and is therefore not made with the usual way. It's not prepared similar to a regular cup of coffee in that it wouldn't suffice to sprinkle water on the beans or on leaves. Ayahuasca is made with highest care and attention to detail and is not made by anybody; a novice can't create it on their own.

It is to be made and simmered under the direction by a wise elder, typically known as a Shaman. The reason for this is that Ayahuasca is crafted by a precise process; the proper quantities of plants and other mixtures should be ensured for a proper variation of the Ayahuasca mix.

Ayahuasca and Shamans share a close relation to each other. The blend of Ayahuasca along with Shaman Shaman will result in greater healing effect that a regular ceremony could result in. Naturally, Ayahuasca is a powerful substance on its own, and has the ability to heal both the body as well as the soul. It is believed that when it is made with the help by an Shaman senior, the outcome is more potent and effective. Many even suggest that, to a degree, the full effect of Ayahuasca can't be achieved when there isn't a Shaman elder during the making and consumption of the beverage.

So, it's strongly recommended that prior to drinking Ayahuasca one should locate an Shaman and speak with the Shaman about which type of Ayahuasca to drink. One should also inquire with the Shaman questions about the results of Ayahuasca in addition to the Shaman will inform them about the effects of it. Shamans are Shamans are, along with those who are a part of the ritual and sacrament of Ayahuasca they are the best informed regarding the drink, particularly for the region that they reside in.

The Shamans possess a wealth of knowledge of healing, as well as the forest. They go through a phase during their training, where they venture into the woods to study the spirits of the plants. They are of the belief that, as humans, trees and plants are spirits and examine which plants have healing properties. Shamans are thought, by some to be able to discern how to achieve spiritual healing. They are thought to have the ability to manage spirits, particularly the spirits of trees and plants. Furthermore, it's Shamans, or Shamans that can read visions that people experience after taking the Ayahuasca. They have the ability to utilize information about the plants as well as spirits to interpret the visions.

That's why that it is extremely recommended to bring an Shaman to guide you throughout your Ayahuasca journey. A Shaman can be able to answer any questions you may have concerning the complete Ayahuasca experience and the intricate procedure. The real Shaman will also assist to identify people who disguise themselves as "Shamans." The real Shamans consider they are "fake" Shamans mislead people looking to take a trip

Ayahuasca typically trying to make a profit from ignorant customers.

Naturally, it is crucial to shield yourself from harm by understanding the history of certain shamans Ayahuasca retreats and Ayahuasca drinks before you dive in.

What to Expect in an Ayahuasca Ceremony?

Prior to the ceremony it is possible to be requested to take a bath with flowers. This helps your appeal, and to connect to the Ayahuasca spirit of the plant. Also, it is recommended to take moments with the plant world in the days prior to your ceremony so that you are able to connect with the "plant consciousness" better.

The Ayahuasca ceremony usually takes place during the night. Darkness is conducive for visions. The beverage makes the eyes more sensitive to the light. If the celebration is in the wilderness, the ceremony begins as it becomes dark when it's in a bustling city it will be delayed until the city is calm.

The shaman stays at the center and the group will create an arc around him, and stand in front of the spiritual leader. This is to bring the focus of energy onto the same spot. Participants can sit on mats or chairs. it is not recommended to lie down as it can be disorienting and can cause people to get sleepy and choke on the urine.

Icaros (shamanic song) are sung in the beginning of the ceremony to welcome spirits. When the participant has sung into the bottle of Ayahuasca and pouring it into participants' cups before handing it over to the participants. In many cases, he'll sing in each cup too.

Once everyone is drank the tea, the lights are turned off and candles set out. Then, the icaros are performed again, along with rattles of leaves also known as Chakapas. Chakapas and icaros direct the flow of energy throughout the area in order to purify, direct as well as protect.

Tobacco plant is believed to be sacred to Shamanic shamans. Smoking tobacco is an option during the Ayahuasca ceremony, which is to cleanse the space of negative spirit and energy, as well as for sealing off the space away from these energies. Shamans can blow smoke over the participant's chest and head or sprinkle it throughout the space using the chakapas, or fan composed of large feathers. Participants may receive tobacco to use for smoking.

The ceremony lasts from between 4 and 6 hours. The Ayahuasca effects last over a period of 2 to six hours. These effects can last from up to eight hours following the most intense feeling. Experiences will differ in accordance with the following factors:

Dosage

Types of substances that are employed

The metabolism of a person

What is the amount and when the individual has ate

Be sure to not drink until the shaman is ready to give the cup over to you. He will present it to you only when he believes that it's the appropriate moment for you to consume the drink.

The Ayahuasca is ayahuasca that kicks in between 20 and 60 minutes after you have consumed it. Be sure not to ask for a drink because there is nothing taking place. Effects may occur after, and should you consume a second glass and the effect intensifies, it may be excessive for your comfort.

Participants will spend some time experiencing the benefits of Ayahuasca. Participants can discuss this as well as other topics with one the other.

The area for the ceremony is considered sacred and is protected by energy. It's not advised to be away from the place for long periods during the course of Ayahuasca. Ayahuasca Ayahuasca stimulates the energetic body and helps you open to the realm of spirit. There is a chance of encountering spirit and negative forces when you leave the safe zone. In addition, the process of taking Ayahuasca is similar to having a moderate dose of alcohol. The risk is that you may fall off balance or even get lost.

Don't eat meals right after drinking Ayahuasca. It will be thrown out. Then wait until noon on the next day to eat something lighter.

It is common response to Ayahuasca and therefore all are encouraged to carry a bucket containers. It is possible to ritually tossing into the earth in a sign of remitting the substance back to soil.

As the event is getting close to end The lights are turned off again. Participants and shamans will engage with one another during this time. People who are exhausted might want to go to sleep.

Chapter 5: Effects

There are numerous claims regarding the results of the consumption of Ayahuasca. Since it's the psychedelic cocktail that has a psychedelic effect, the effects will be evident to everyone who consumes the drink. That means that, unlike the other drugs and plants which can be ingested Ayahuasca is almost sure to produce some form of impact on the individual.

As with every other psychedelic there are positive as well as positive claims regarding the results of consumption of Ayahuasca. There are some assertions that the results of Ayahuasca last for a long time; however other people claim that it is only a short-term effect. Regarding the time of the effects, it's typically safe to conclude that the more potent the Ayahuasca mix is, the greater its effects are. The time of the effects will also be contingent upon the amount of alcohol consumed by the individual, in addition to the ingredients used.

Regarding the positive experience Some people who've taken Ayahuasca claim that they had some revelations concerning their mission within the world. A few have even claimed that they realized the truth of the earth as well as the universe via their experiences. Another common positive experience is individuals recognizing how to become the most effective person they could be and what they should be doing in taking care of others. This is the result of expanding one's awareness that allows them to see their world free of the self-concept they've built up over time.

Regarding negative experience, the argument is that since it's a remedy that has purging properties It can cleanse the body through diarrhoea and vomiting. hallucinations are also a possible result of Ayahuasca since the drink is a source of hallucinogens. Many consider this to be an adverse effect some are afraid to accept this truth. But, even though it contains a variety of exotic substances, there's currently no study in the scientific literature that could lead to Ayahuasca being classed as an "dangerous drug."

It's important to be aware that, prior to and foremost Ayahuasca's primary function is as a healing drug. It's only natural that it could have numerous impacts on human bodies. Below is what you must be aware of the benefits of Ayahuasca and how they can be achieved.

Before discussing the benefits of Ayahuasca be helpful to briefly review the various levels of brainwaves:

Beta (12 Hz - 40 Hz):

A normal state of consciousness that permits rational thinking. It's most commonly seen in the case of a person who is performing some activity.

Alpha (8Hz - 12 Hz):

Relaxation is a state of mind. It occurs when a individual is daydreaming or imagining some thing, contemplating or is near to falling to sleep.

Theta (4 Hz - 8 Hz):

A state of trance that is deep. It is when a person connects to their unconscious mind and feelings. In this state, people are susceptible to the hypnotic effects. Theta usually occurs during the night, but one may experience it through the practice of meditation, or through taking the trance-producing substances like Ayahuasca.

The Delta (lower than four Hz):

The person is unable to sleep and has no dreams. This happens when someone has fallen asleep, or if he or she suffers trauma to the brain or has a mental illness.

Based on a study conducted with 12 volunteers at the Ayahuasca workshops in Brazil Drinking Ayahuasca tea can increase theta and alpha brainwaves. After 3 doses of tea, the participants' EEG readings showed significant rises in the frequency and frequency of their Alpha (8-13 HZ) and theta (4-8 4-8 Hz) brainwaves. The increase of alpha waves was observed within the occipital lobes and the rise in theta wave frequency was seen in the frontal and occipital lobes.

The evidence suggests that those who drink Ayahuasca can experience a state of consciousness, which is higher than the normal reflection state. The state of trance permits them to connect with their subconscious and remain in a state of consciousness.

Physiological Effects

Beware; the Ayahuasca beverage has a bitter flavor. It's oily, bitter and viscous. It is possible to gag when drinking it.

Ayahuasca is widely recognized as the purging chemical that is a psychedelic. It purifies the body through inducing it to eliminate unnecessary chemicals. The Ayahuasca mix has the result that can cause nausea and diarrhea for some however not all users. It is a good thing that people can to feel the full benefits of the Ayahuasca drink, regardless of regardless of whether they vomit up.

The Emetic (vomit-inducing) as well as the purgative (diarrhea-inducing) consequences of harmaline are lessen as your body becomes accustomed to the harmaline. The hallucinogenic impact doesn't seem to diminish in the case of experienced users.

Ayahuasca could also lead to an impairment to a person's motor capabilities, because it alters certain motor functions in the brain. But this specific impact isn't lasting in accordance with studies that have been conducted. Motor skills are impaired will only last for a brief and brief period following the consumption of the drink.

DMT which is inhaled or injection, can have immediate effects. They usually last just 30 minutes. Orally consumed Ayahuasca can take a long time to take in, and yet it lasts for as long as up to 4-6 hours.

The eyes can become sensitive to light when Ayahuasca is in action within the body. That's why it is often very dimly illuminated. Avoid looking at sources of light that are bright for instance, the moment you see someone else is smoking cigarettes.

Psychological Effects

A lot of people who have attempted Ayahuasca say that there is some kind of effect on their minds after they drink the beverage. Most commonly, they say following the consumption of Ayahuasca visions begin appearing in a flash. At first, visions appear mixed colors, and then after a while they become more vivid. These colors create different curves and lines, and transform into stunning.

In the end, these various shapes will form an exact picture. The image or group of pictures is based on what those who have consumed Ayahuasca is able to be reflecting. Furthermore to this, the auditory and tactile senses of an individual are more sensitive.

Also, their mental state is thought to be greater.

Although the majority of people claim that this is the case however, there are certain people who believe that there wasn't an amazing visual display. They say they observed a small visual display that was a mix of color and light. Some even that have experienced horrific events with Ayahuasca that included insomnia and a little sleep paralysis. This isn't as frequent, and is even rarer in the presence by Shamans. Shaman.

The effect that occurs from Ayahuasca which is distinctive in psychedelics is that it has the ability to bring deep-seated parts of the mind to come to the surface. It allows one to comprehend the thoughts, and in some cases, amaze themselves with insight that was not readily accessible to them in a ordinary state of mind. Many practitioners believe that its purgative effects are a symbol of the letting go of mental pressures.

Spiritual Effect

A lot of people who have drank Ayahuasca reported that they experienced a sense of enlightenment after taking the drink. The people who have testified, actually it was as if they had found the purpose of their lives. Others also claim they found something to be thankful for in their lives, when they previously had no or meaning. After drinking, they experienced a sense like a rebirth. This is why Ayahuasca can be quite effective for people that feel like they've hit a brick wall when they try to achieve their goals or who have been in a rut emotionally.

The effect of spirituality of a person can be enough to make them feel a necessity to modify their lifestyles and routines. The theory is that this is due to the cathartic experience, and this response will be stronger when Shaman. Shaman.

Possible Benefits of Ayahuasca

Altered Perspective

There is a chance to change your perception of what is happening around your. It is possible to see things in a completely different way from a different perspective.

Enhanced Imagination

It is possible to enter the space of your imagination where you'll experience the imagined world in real life. Your enhanced imagination to perform a wide range of different things.

Enhanced Creativity

Your imagination could grow significantly, as you'll be connected to the part of your brain that is able to generate innovative thoughts. It's like you were a kid once more. The limitations of life disappear and it is possible to rekindle your passions you've been suppressing.

Psychic Visions

Visions will pop up. They may come out of the depths of your mind. However, others could come from different sources. They could provide useful insights that you can use for your own life.

Profound Realizations

It is possible to learn new things. Then you will get a fresh view of things you are familiar with. It will also cause you to rethink things that seemed to make sense previously to you.

Self-Improvement

Self-improvement, whether it's getting something you want or shedding undesirable traits is much easier in a state of mind that Ayahuasca induces. It is better to change old habits performed in a other environment because Ayahuasca breaks patterns of thought and the automatic responses. Apart from that, Ayahuasca creates positive feelings and increases the willpower of a person.

Connecting with the Divine

Shamans believe in Ayahuasca as a way of connecting our human brain to the mind of an ethereal living being. It is believed to be aware of its own. It is believed to be a powerful spiritual being that is capable of healing and guiding individuals.

Characteristics of the Ayahuasca Spirit:

Divine

Sentient

Caring

Loving

Powerful

Feminine

Playful

Understanding

Wise

Sensual

The way people perceive Ayahuasca in different ways. Ayahuasca Spirit differently. It is possible to be amazed in the manner it reveals its self for you.

Healing at Various Levels

Ayahuasca is considered to be a holy medicine for the mind, body, and spirit. It's said to have the ability to regulate the biochemistry of your body. It helps to heal the mind by bringing the suppressed parts to the forefront, ensuring that you are able to deal with them successfully. You become conscious of your soul's existence and brings you closer to God. That's why many would be willing to sacrifice in exchange for Ayahuasca.

Purgation

The physical manifestations of diarrhea and vomiting are symptoms to eliminate harmful substances from the body, mind and the soul. Avoid forcing yourself to throw up when you don't desire to do so. The belief is that when you allow the Ayahuasca "tell" you when to vomit, it can clear the negative energy and blocks within your. If you also puke excessively and in a hurry your body could not be able to take in the Ayahuasca therefore your experiences won't be as powerful.

Chapter 6: Ayahuasca Ceremony Preparations

Physical Preparation

In order to protect yourself, you must ensure you're physically fit enough to consume Ayahuasca. It will be helpful if you get a medical clearance/certificate before going into the ceremony or drinking the brew on your own. It will provide an assurance that you'll be okay regardless of whether you drank the most potent brew that induces hallucinations.

If you are suffering from any of the ailments the best option is not to take Ayahuasca. The consumption of Ayahuasca can be stressful for the body. Additionally, the treatment for the conditions may interact adversely to the Ayahuasca drinks ingredients. Particularly, the interactions between the two could result in blocking nerve transmitters that control blood pressure. This means that it could rise to levels that are dangerous, resulting in a stroke or heart attack.

Also, think about getting better prior to seeking your physician's recommendations if you are suffering from any of one of the following ailments:

Prescription medications (especially MAOIs SSRIs and vasodilators, as well as antihypertensives, asthma medications and appetite suppressants CNS depression medications, as well as antipsychotics). Interactions between drugs and Ayahuasca are addressed further on.

Heart disease:

Ayahuasca can cause the heartbeat to be faster and more vigorously.

Blood pressure that is low or high:

Patients with blood pressure issues are at risk of the physiological effects of Ayahuasca.

Asthma, for example: asthma

Ayahuasca could cause exhaustion for people with breathing issues.

Kidney disease and/or liver:

If your kidneys or liver are in trouble this means that the body will be incapable of eliminating the toxic and harmful substances inside the body.

Intestinal ulcers:

Ayahuasca consumption is fasting-related; the result is that ulcers are worsened.

Allergies:

The brew's allergens or any other drink could cause harm to your health.

The blood sugar and diabetes-related illnesses:

Food is not consumed throughout ceremonies like the Ayahuasca ceremony. Diarrhea and vomiting are also possible. This can cause the blood sugar level to drop. levels. If you suffer from this disorder drinking fruit in the morning and during the ceremony can aid in managing your illness.

Mental illness (manic-depressive and psychosis Clinical depression):

Ayahuasca could help in curing mental disorders, but it can cause them to get more severe. People with suicidal tendencies could be harmed while being under the influence of Ayahuasca.

Epilepsy and various seizure disorders:

The effects of Ayahuasca increase the brain's electrical stimulation and could trigger seizures. Additionally, it can hinder the effectiveness of medications that prevent seizures.

Anesthetics are required for medical procedures (surgery and dental procedure):

The MAOIs present in Ayahuasca could increase the intensity of the effects of anesthetics and can create problems. You should wait at least two weeks after clearing before you drink Ayahuasca.

The effects of breastfeeding and pregnancies:

The mother of a baby who is pregnant must avoid using substances that aren't safe for infants, as they can also be eaten by the child. It is possible to reconsider Ayahuasca if you've already had your baby and quit nursing.

Warning:

The inhibition of MAO-A (monoamine oxidase) enzymes can cause an rise in neurotransmitters including norephinephrine, dopamine and melatonin. tryptamine, as well as other amines. Tetrahydroharmine stops the breakdown of serotonin as well. This can lead to a number of issues like:

Hypertensive Crisis (sharp increase in blood pressure which may cause a heart attack or stroke)

Serotonin syndrome (symptoms include agitation, a rapid heart rate, irregular heartbeat, hypertension and seizures, as well as high fever Shivering, diarrhea muscles twitching/loss coordination (symptoms:

headache, disorientation and loss of consciousness)

Psychosis

The blockade of MAO could also result in the overproduction of epinephrine as well as norepineph that could lead to:

Angina (intense chest pain)

Confusion

Eye damage

Heart attack

Hypertensive crisis (rapid increasing of blood pressure)

Kidney problems

Memory loss

Migraine

Edema of the lungs (accumulation of fluids within the lung)

Unconsciousness

Apart from that in addition, a dopamine/levodopa (L-dopa) dose can also result in psychosis as well as the signs that are associated with anxiety and confusion. It can also cause delusions, confusion as well as hallucinations.

Due to these dangers It is vital that you follow these rules before taking Ayahuasca:

The Diet

The diet prescribed is for those who take Ayahuasca. It is made up of a foods that have been proven that over time, not cause any adverse effects after consumption with the Ayahuasca plant.

The diet is a way to cleanse the body of energetic and physical impureties. It is essential to adhere to the diet in order to prevent any issues when you participate in ceremony. Ayahuasca ceremony.

Consume healthy foods, such as raw food, fresh vegetables as well as fruits, and also juices made from vegetables.

Reduce the consumption of red meats like venison, pork and duck from 1 week to 6 months prior to the ceremony. It takes longer for meat to digest. Also, it is believed that animal flesh has "negative energies" by some Shamans due to how it's prepared. The Ayahuasca can force dirty and undigested food from the body. Hence, ensure that your meals prior to the ceremony can be digested easily.

Do not consume chocolates, caffeine as well as other stimulants that include stimulant Amino acids.

It is equally essential to not eat foods or substances which react to MAOIs for at minimum 3 days prior to consuming Ayahuasca. Some examples of this are tyramine-containing products, like:

Alcohol

Aged foods (aged cheese and aged meat)

Banana peels

Beans (some species, such as broad bean pods Italian Green beans, Fava beans snow peas)

Beer

Brewer's yeast (baker's yeast works fine)

Dry fruits

Incorrectly stored poultry, meat as well as fish that has been improperly stored

Kimchee

Malts

Overripe fruit

Food that is picked

Rich food

Sauerkraut

Shrimp paste

Smoked meat

Soybean products (soy sauce, fermented soya beans, etc.)

Wines

Extracts of yeast (Vegemite, Marmite)

The least risky option, however to avoid

Avocados

Bananas

Bouillon (beef or chicken)

Caffeine (in safe doses)

Cheeses (cream cheese, cottage cheese, ricotta, processed)

Chocolate

Fish (fresh and uncooked, or smoked or picked)

Meat (fresh)

Monosodium glutamate (MSG)

Peanuts

Poultry

Raspberries

Beware of spicy food. If you consume them before purgative can cause discomfort.

Beware of unhealthy foods like processed, fried or oily foods, sweets and unhealthy food items for a month prior to the ceremony. (Ayahuasca can cleanse the body of toxins. Help in the cleansing process by avoiding food items that aren't good to your health).

Do not eat a heavy meal during the time of the ceremony. Drinking water or juices of fruit for a drink to quench your thirst.

Drug - Ayahuasca Interactions

REMEMBER:

Consult your physician regarding the possibility of taking Ayahuasca. Discuss if it is possible to put off taking the medicine for a time so that you can avoid adverse drug-ayahuasca interactions. If your physician isn't happy with your Ayahuasca consumption, you should consider seeking a second opinion, or stopping your Ayahuasca strategies.

If a few medical professionals tell you that Ayahuasca can be very harmful for you, do not be surprised. Ayahuasca increases the impact of DMT. The pineal gland makes this substance in the natural course of the night, and particularly in meditative and dream states. It is possible to try meditation or learning to lucidly dream as an alternative. The same but more secure, results.

In addition there are other drug classes to look out for

Antidepressants (Do not wait six weeks prior to consuming Ayahuasca)

DARI

NARI

NaSSA

NRI

SNDRI

SNRI

SSRE

SSRI

TCA

TeCa

Some prescription drugs can cause interactions with Ayahuasca (avoid drinking for two weeks before drinking the beverage If possible):

ADHD medications

Amitryptamine

Amoxipine

Amphetamines

Anesthetics

Anti-allergy meds

Antihistamines

Antinarcoleptic medication

Antipsychotics

Appetite suppressants

Asthma medication

Barbiturates

Benzodiapines

Medicines to lower blood pressure (high blood pressure) or blood pressure that is low)

Cold medications

Meds for diabetes

Diuretics

Meds for the flu

Heart medications

L-dopa containing meds

The effects of muscle relaxants

Opioids

Painkillers

Seizure meds

Sinus medication

Sleep pills

Vasodilators

All drugs that have adverse side effects when combined together with MAOIs

The recreational drug (Avoid during the 6-8 weeks preceding Ayahuasca consumption)

It's not recommended to use recreational drugs in the beginning and after, Ayahuasca use. The drugs could contain chemicals that pose danger when used in conjunction with the ingredients of Ayahuasca. In addition the herbs that are used in Ayahuasca are considered sacred.

Alcohol

Amphetamines

Barbiturates

Caffeine (recreational use in large amounts)

Cannabis

Cocaine

Codeine

Dexamphetamine

Dissociative anesthetics

DMT

DXM/DM/DX (dextromethorphan)

Ephedrine

Ergo lines

Heroin

Kava

Ketamine

Kratom

LSA

LSD

Lysergamides

MDA

MDEA

MDMA (ecstasy)

Mescaline

Methadone

Methamphetamine

Morphine

Nutmeg

Opiates

Opium

PCP

Phenethylamine

PMA

Psilocin

Psilocybin

Sedatives

Shrooms

Tryptamines

5-MEO-DMT

Enhancers of energy (Don't take them for 1 day before taking Ayahuasca)

Consuming energy boosters made with Ayahuasca is a drain on your energy levels and create strain in your heart. A few of them are as the following:

Ephedra

Ginseng

Kava

Rhodiola

Sinicuichi

Yohimbe

Energy drinks

Mood Enhancers (Avoid one day before)

Ayahuasca can alter the brain's chemical chemistry mood boosters, and any other substances that do the same can cause confusion and even harm. Examples include:

Ephedra

Inositol

Kava

L-Theanine

Rhodiola

SAMe

St. John's Wort

Tyramine/Tryptophan (Avoid one day before)

Protein powders

Exercise supplements

Sleep Aids (Avoid 1 day prior)

Kava

Melatonin

Dopamine and Norepinephrine (Avoid one day before)

5-HTP

L-DOPA

L-Phenylalanine

L-tryptophan

L-tyrosine

Psychological Preparation

Intention

It is essential to enter the ceremony with a seriousness and an explicit purpose for performing this. It is suggested that you create a plan to the ceremony based on the following reasons:

For the best enjoyment of your Experience

In order to direct your thinking

For you to increase your determination

to prevent you from becoming lost in a Trance

to appreciate the significance of the ritual

Allow Ayahuasca's spirit to interact with you. Ayahuasca to connect with you.

It should be a simple goal and you won't be able to overlook it in the course, particularly in times of intense tension. Make it a short, simple mantra. It should be easy to quickly repeat the mantra.

Some examples of the ideal intentions:

"I request healing"

"I seek guidance"

"I want clarity","I'm looking for clarity,.

Spiritual Practice

The practice of a spiritual life isn't required, however it's a good way to increase the degree of satisfaction you have. Meditation, for instance or pranic healing as well as qi gong, tai Chi as well as yoga will enable you to lead your mind into the psychedelic world which will allow you to control the energy you meet in that realm.

Mindfulness

It can benefit you significantly if developed the ability to pay at the present as well as the events which happen in the world around your. When you are accustomed to this type of awareness it will allow you to take into the Ayahuasca experiences and have many more of the memories of what might occur to the person you are. You'll be able to see more visions, as well as gain lots of information because of it.

Emotional Control

Controlling your emotions is important as Ayahuasca amplifies feelings and triggers images which are then based upon them. This also stops the person from becoming anxious. Here are a few methods that can help you manage your emotions:

Clearing your mind

Concentrating on the intention

Relaxing

Deep-breathing

The memory of an experience which brings about a desire emotion

Smiling

Singing a mantra that can make you feel great

Being observant of emotions without judging them

The analysis of emotion

Expressing emotion through communication

Paying no attention to emotional state, instead you are distracted by another thing

Doing everything to make the emotion go away

Not Interrupting Others

While you might go through the ceremony with other people, each one has their own experience. Do your best not to disrupt others as you are experiencing your visions. Don't help the person, even if you feel you should be able to, unless you are sure they're being threatened.

There is a chance that they may have to endure certain uncomfortable experiences to gain some valuable information or recover from a condition. Do your best to not keep them distracted from the task at hand by focusing on your own personal experiences rather.

Not Resisting the Experience

As you experience Ayahuasca's effects, try to not be averse to what you feel. Refusing to accept it can increase the severity of it, since when you're feeling negatively about what's going on, that negativity will manifest within the images.

That's why you're advised to concentrate on the positive aspects of life. Remind yourself of your objectives and keep in mind these. Think of everything that happens as an opportunity to heal the need to experience.

Sex and Masturbation

According to a few shamans Ayahuasca ceremonies participants are advised to stay clear of masturbation or sexual contact up to a week prior the ceremony is scheduled to take place.

The reasons for this are:

In order to stop the transmission of subtle energies between an individual, who could affect one's energy field.

In order to conserve your own energie and to dedicate it to the ceremony.

Ayahuasca is a spirit of the desert. Ayahuasca spirit is thought to be jealous of lovers, that is dissatisfied with sexually attractive individuals.

Abstinence can give you powerful dreams.

This is a way that involves "sublimating" your sexual energy or changing it into spiritual energy.

Elimination from Vices

Abstaining from vices and "energetically-unclean" activities and substances will lessen the things that Ayahuasca will purge from you. According to shamans, it will enhance Ayahuasca's spiritual benefits.

Things to Bring:

There are the following during the course of your Ayahuasca trip:

Mattress

Pillows

Yoga chair

Sleeping bag

Shawls, blankets, or even blankets

Bottles for water and Thermos - Used for storing juice, water and tea

Container or bucket in which you can throw away

Tissue

Toiletries

Sunblock lotion

Bug repellent

Clothing (preferably lighter-colored because they are believed to attract positive spirits. On the contrary those with dark colors are believed to attract evil spirits)

Long sleeved sweaters/shirts

Comfy pants

Shorts

Hat

Swimsuit

Hiking boots

Sandals

Eye masks - These are designed to protect your eyes from light sources particularly when you're getting ready going to bed. Additionally, wearing an eye-mask on can aid in focusing on your images.

Flashlight (ideally coated by red cellophane in order to prevent eye injuries) The ritual is to be conducted in darkness.

Batteries

Chapter 7: Ayahuasca And Other Psychedelics

The psychedelics belong to the category of active drugs that are also known as hallucinogens. These substances are capable on the way of thinking and perception of the individual who is taking their. The reason that psychedelics are so sought-after is due to the fact that the psychedelic compounds cause an euphoria that creates a dream-like experience inside the brain as well as body. It is possible to experience dreams that do not exist physically However, they appear to be real for the brain.

Additionally, psychedelic drugs are able to enhance the senses of the person. The smallest details of something even a person with average perception won't be able to see, are visible for someone who is taking a psychedelic. They become more receptive also, particularly to bright colors and lights. The effects described above, taken as a total, also are results of an Ayahuasca mixture. While they might vary in intensity and duration, the resemblances can be seen. There are, however, certain key distinctions:

The first thing to note is that people who consume Ayahuasca feel nauseated and more likely be prone to vomit. While some believe that a badly made Ayahuasca can cause vomiting and nausea it is important to note the fact that Ayahuasca can be described as a cleansing drink It is common that people throw up. Its primary function is to eliminate harmful substances from your body. This is why it causes dizziness and nausea it's effective in achieving that goal. Many psychedelics don't usually possess the same impact. Most commonly, drugs for psychedelics aren't used to cause nausea. Certain people might experience a small amount of nausea. However, it's due to its effect on cognition and perception of the person.

The second is that a lot of people who take Ayahuasca is seeking for a spiritual effects. If they are looking to be rejuvenated, discover their purpose to live their lives or determine the purpose of their lives, many consider that because they're participating in a sacred ceremony, there's an unknown force or energy that helps people to experience the same. However, this isn't as it is with other drugs that are psychedelic. Most often, someone who takes psychedelics knows that chances of experiencing some positive spiritual effects is minimal or no at all. Most of the time it is because the reason to take the psychedelics you're taking is to be taken to a new reality. This is often employed as a way that allows you to leave the humdrum of life within the normal day and be transported to a world that is awash with light and color.

Thirdly, Ayahuasca requires a sacred ceremony. Most people who drink Ayahuasca don't believe it's an authentic Ayahuasca experience when there's no sense of sacredness in the experience, be it be at the preparation phase or the stage of drinking; however psychoactive substances do not generally feature this attribute. For many, they are merely a way to induce a different reality but they are not sacred and spiritual instruments.

The last, Ayahuasca, alone, is generally considered to be as legal. It is legal in the United States, Ayahuasca is considered a valid beverage, tea, and mix. The plant itself isn't harmful for well-being. Additionally, the plant and herbs that are typically used to create Ayahuasca are not classified as illicit, neither. Only when Ayahuasca is a controlled substance that it is considered illegal. In contrast certain other psychedelics are classified as harmful substances and are legally unlawful.

Chapter 8: Ayahuasca Today

Today, Ayahuasca still maintains its popularity as an ancient healing remedy that has a long history. A lot of celebrities, including Lindsay Lohan, for example are turning to the Ayahuasca journey with the goal to resolve the chaos in their lives. Another benefit that Ayahuasca is considered to have to be effective in the present it's ability to aid in the recovery of any addiction to substances, no matter if related to alcohol or drugs. While this hasn't yet been scientifically tested however, there are instances where people were able to break the habit completely, by using Ayahuasca.

Another benefit of Ayahuasca is that, even in the modern world it serves to ease stress and anxiety when you have enough resources. In the midst of all the pressure that everyone is subjected to as well as all the negative energy and negative vibes that the contemporary life can generate, some users try Ayahuasca in order to lessen or eliminate stress that come with daily living.

A different context is Ayahuasca is being utilized as a way to increase tourism in different regions of South America. Due to the long-standing indigenous, sacred, and native ritual that the Ayahuasca experiences the experience to be fascinating for many across the globe. People of South America use this to encourage curious visitors to their country to try Ayahuasca. In light of the fact that there are a myriad of questionable elements in the Ayahuasca experience, until one is able to experience the experience of drinking Ayahuasca and is able to understand its purpose by studying about it.

It's not just tourists, persons who plan to see the Shamans Researchers and scientists are making trips to these countries too. Due to the increasing interest in Ayahuasca and its benefits, people are eager to understand why it functions in the way it does. Scientists are looking into the various substances and their effect upon the human brain. It is possible that there are healing qualities from plants which could aid in curing various diseases that we're currently struggling as a nation.

Chapter 9: Legality

The intense effects of Ayahuasca and its effects, especially those like those found in other psychedelic drugs as well as controlled substances, have caused many to doubt the lawfulness of this sacred remedy. Can it be classified as an illicit drug?

In the past, as I've mentioned In America, in the United States, it is legal to possess the Ayahuasca plant, also called the Banisteriopsis Caapi inside one's house. It is, however, not legal to consume the grapevine to enjoy leisure or recreational reasons. As it's considered to be as a sacred drug it is believed to be a sacred medicine. Ayahuasca vine can be used to pursue the practice of religious convictions. But it's not necessarily legal to possess. Anyone who wants to take ayahuasca drink Ayahuasca has to first provide the evidence that proves it's being used to fulfill religious reasons.

Furthermore, if Ayahuasca vine is paired with plants or other herbs which do not belong to the classification of Schedule-I and Schedule-I, then one is able to drink it legal. Drugs that fall under Schedule-I are thought to be a risk to cause harm, and have been proven to provide no health benefits whatsoever. What does fall into this classification are Di-Methyl Triptamine, more commonly referred to as DMT. If DMT is used as an ingredient to Ayahuasca this concoction turns into illegal. The concoction is at this time, subject to oversight and supervision that is the responsibility of United States Government.

As a result, a lot of Shamans throughout America United States, now, are taking care when it comes to the preparation and giving of Ayahuasca. They're putting out warnings so that they can comply with the regulations of the state and are advising regarding the use of Ayahuasca consumed by women who are pregnant or anyone suffering from heart disease. Even though the legality of these mixtures is not clear, Shamans still prefer to make the appropriate precautions to maintain their trustworthiness.

Positively, even though Ayahuasca concoctions can be deemed unlawful in certain circumstances however, there are some authorities who do not care regarding it. They are of the opinion that drug-related incidents are more serious and risky than those involving Ayahuasca. They prefer to handle situations that have been proven to be risky to individuals, rather than tampering with the healing ceremonies associated with Ayahuasca.

International Laws

Brazil

Brazil has been legalizing Ayahausca as well as the other plants associated with it in 1992. In the 1980s, there were legal disputes between Ayahuasca users and the authorities which ended when it was discovered that using Ayahuasca during religious ceremonies doesn't cause harm to anyone.

France

It is illegal to consume Ayahuasca to be consumed in France. In in 2005 France is announcing the following substances as controlled:

Banisteriopsis caapi

Banisteriopsis rusbyana

Mimosa hostiles

Psychotria Viridis

Peganum harmala

Harmaline

Harmine

Tetrahydroharmine

Psychotria viridis

Diplopterys

Peganum harmala

Netherlands

Ayahuasca is legally legal within the Netherlands. It's typically offered in the smart shop or in stores selling psychoactive (mind-altering) drugs.

Canada

Harmaline is an Schedule III drug in Canada. Ayahuasca beverages usually contain harmaline. It is therefore likely to be considered to be illegal to drink the brews.

Spain

Ayahuasca isn't regulated in Spain.

United Kingdom

Ayahuasca is banned in the UK since it is a source of DMT that is classified as a drug.

United States

Ayahuasca as well as DMT plants are typically legal. However, DMT is an illegal Schedule I drug.

United Nations

As per the United Nations Drug Control Program the DMT-containing plants do not fall in the international drug control program.

Some Tips Regarding Legality & Location

Know about Ayahuasca laws in your region.

Make sure the seller is in possession of A Privacy Policy.

Avoid travel in a vehicle that contains Ayahuasca in brewed or plant in its brewed.

Chapter 10: Costs

Despite the fact that Ayahuasca originates from combination of various plants and herbs It isn't cheap to experience the Ayahuasca experiencing. It is possible to find the forests, in the wilderness, or even to certain people the backyard are herbs as well as plants. But what's priced to the customer is the whole experience not just the herb or plants.

The entire experience typically is accompanied by a discussion of what Ayahuasca blend is the best one for the individual as well as the making of the mixture with the help of Shaman Shaman as well as the ritual of drinking as well as the evaluation of the results.

The entire ceremony typically, the price ranges between $150-$350. It includes one evening of the Ayahuasca experience. The drink is made up of between ten and twelve cups Ayahuasca. Some areas provide packages ranging between $650 and $2,000 according to the content of the bundles. Price also varies based on the length of the guest's stay. Some would prefer to extend their stay in the event of an optimistic view of the experience.

Certain packages might include a treatment experience at a retreat, a healing session or other additional services. Retreats provide place to stay for the individual who is taking advantage of this package. The retreat could last 3-7 days, dependent on the type of Ayahuasca experiences the person is looking for. The experience of healing is, however is more dependent to what the Shaman and the kind of services they can offer.

Ayahuasca can, at times, be accessible from underground stores as well as "smart shops" at approximately 50 dollars per dosage. Anahuasca (Ayahuasca Analogues) generally cost less than Ayahuasca produced from B. caapi, and P. viridis.

Whatever your budget or the kind of plan you're looking at, the main thing is to be sure that you've done your study prior to making any decision. It is important to find someone that can provide you with an opinion, and choose a reliable Shaman to change the satisfaction. When you've paid for the service for the service, you shouldn't worry over whether you're receiving the correct quality of service. Instead, you should be focused on the overall experience, and relying on the Shaman.

Chapter 11: Tips Before Beginning The Ayahuasca Diet

What are the best ways to prepare to experience Ayahuasca? There's no way to predict what to be expecting from your very first excursion. But, you'll be prepared in the event that you've had previous psychoactive experiences and know the risks and the best way to protect yourself.

Getting in Shape

Human bodies are in fact the vessel. Every thing we do to our bodies--the meals we eat, our ideas we have or the exercises we perform leaves an impression. Our surroundings' materials influence us physically, but also psychologically, emotionally, as well as spiritually.

If you think about the vessel that which you travel with all over the world Your body, too, is an element of your energy system. It receives and transmits energy. It's an integral part of everything in existence. It serves like a filter that absorbs. Due to the substances it absorbs it can become clogged or blocked, even overwhelmed. If not addressed and untreated, the effect on this negative energy could be disastrous. That's why it's so important to ensure optimal levels of hygiene within your body in order to ensure the highest quality of energy exchange between your body and its environment.

But, if we exercise your due diligence and read our bodies and minds for experiencing the Ayahuasca experience, we open the path for the Ayahuasca experience to better connect to us and achieve its purposes. While perfection is not possible but you must still try the best you can in order to be more prepared.

Mental Tune-Up

What you put into the body is equally vital as what you put inside your head while taking the ayahuasca diet. The preparation of the mind and body to experience the journey could have positive results along with the physical cleansing process that takes place through the entire process.

In the days leading up to your retreat, try to ensure that your mind is as clear of anxiety as you can by keeping your distance from undesirable people or events. Spend a few days off prior to the event to rest, meditate and focus on your goal within the nature with no distractions of technology. If that's not possible, then it is best to reduce the amount of time you are on the couch as well as using social media.

Sexual Activity

Beware of sexual activity in the weeks leading to the wedding. While plant remedies do their jobs, they're safeguarded, nurtured and governed by the energy reserves in each one of us. Sexual contact in all forms such as the exchange of bodily fluids can be highly charged and will drain your energy resources and reduce the efficacy of the plant medicine in its education role.

What Time of Day Should I Start the Ayahuasca Diet?

If you're considering for a retreat, commence this regimen at least 4 weeks prior to the date. In order to maximize your effectiveness, stay on the diet for at least an additional week after your retreat has ended.

Importantness to The Ayahuasca diet

Here's what you need to know. It is well-known that individuals and the food we eat with can have an enormous impact on the way we live our lives. Your present life depends on your choices and the relationships you have with.

You chose Ayahuasca as you believed you were in need of answers to your toughest concerns. It is a guarantee that Ayahuasca can provide you with unique experiences that assist you in achieving your goals.

Ayahuasca is a potent herbal medicine that operates at a level of physiological function to detect what needs to be eliminated from the body. It's the reason they call her "la purga," and this is also the reason why following the right diet is crucial.

It's possible that you've committed to 4 nights of ritual and you've compiled an agenda of questions you want the Ayahuasca shaman. If you do not adhere strictly to your Ayahuasca food plan, then you could end up spending the greater portion of your time flushing the body of toxic energy or poisons that are affixed to the body.

There may be a slight sort of purging when you adhere to the Ayahuasca diet plan, but this is not as severe as the intense purging that could be experienced if you break the guidelines of your diet.

We're not here to enforce limits, however we wish, along with all of our hearts, that you are having a great time.

We invite you to dedicate your next two weeks being aware of the items you handle and the way they make you feel. You will be able to appreciate your brain as well as Ayahuasca, your mind Spirit of Ayahuasca and the road you're about to set onto.

PREPARING FOR AYAHUASCA RITUAL

How to Prepare Spiritually

The dieta offers guidelines that will help with emotional, mental and spiritual preparation during the weeks leading up to your participation using Ayahuasca. Madre Ayahuasca. The ayahuasqueros of the past would go through the forest on lengthy alone retreats, allowing them to search for and eat vegetation. They would rely only on hunter-gatherer skills. For villages, this could consist of ensuring complete seclusion as well as the restriction of idle chat. The modern diet in advanced countries would certainly include an abstinence from television or radio, movie or news media.

The ideal is to devote at least a few days prior to the ceremony, doing things like meditation, yoga, prayers, mindfulness as well as solitary walks through the forest. Start a conversation of spirituality with Nature prior to your night out with her. Madre is able to open the doors of the direct contact with Pachamama.

What are the reasons to Avoid Negative Vibes when using Ayahuasca Purify

Ayahuasca is an ancient shamanic treatment. Apart from being a powerful mix of psychotropic chemicals that are typically consumed in the form of a ritual container, in which the shaman calls spirits such as ancestral spirits and animal spirits as well as elemental spirits, etc. - to visit the location and help individuals. Spiritually speaking it is believed that the person who drinks ayahuasca can increase the capacity of their mind to perceive and interact with the non-embodied world.

The non-embodied are always evident in Amazonian Shamanism. The belief that in the Amazon that all people are associated with an entourage of spirits that are connected to them. Certain spirits are demons or parasites and often are tied to addiction. Certain are even spiritual. Others are guides, guardians as well as the ancestors.

They can also pick during the normal routine. When your energy fields are wide open, like it is when you are participating in an ayahuasca-related ceremony these beings could "get in" and cause destruction in your life either through illness or misfortune. For a general rule of thumb is to remain at a high vibration and stay clear of getting lost in the"bad part" of town and hanging out at pubs or other places with bad notoriety, or socializing with unsavory people. If you're not able to keep clear of certain locations and places, build up your protection by a more spiritually-focused practice.

Ayahuasca and Sex: Why Should You Avoid Sex Before Attending an Ayahuasca Ceremony?

The two main factors in all Ayahuasca dieta suggestions are to avoid sexual contact and from alcohol. Sexual intimacy is an energetic exchange. If you have been sexually engaged during the time before the ceremony You will likely feel their energy on your energy field very strongly throughout the ceremony. This can be confusing. You may focus more on the person you are with and your relationship than it is. This could result in you feeling more emotionally connected. The person you've had a an intimate relationship with, suddenly appears to be "The One "...

It is when you have sexual fantasies of other persons.

In addition, sexual activity can reduce the amount of energy available to you during the ceremony, which can limit your depth of understanding to where you are able to go psychoanalytically as well as limiting the capacity of your plant to help your journey. It is for this reason that it is recommended to stay clear of masturbation.

The ayahuasca ritual, at every event, is about the spiritual healing process and your personal growth. Therefore it is imperative to keep your energy as pure restricted, secure, and clear from other people as you can.

Chapter 12: Alcohol And Ayahuasca

To date, nobody has passed away due to the combination of alcohol with the ayahuasca. A few of the traditional Ayahuasqueros I've had the privilege of working with was said to take moonshine with cups of ayahuasca in the ceremony. The ayahuasca these people typically drink is extremely mild. This could be the reason that can make this combination even more feasible.

Alcoholism, as with Native Americans in North America are a devastating legacy of colonization, which continues until the present. This older man, the eighth generation of ayahuasqueros from his family, has lived for long periods of time in the solitary dieta the forests and has mastered the art in the limeza. However He is a bit happy with his trago.

Even though Ayahuasca and alcohol aren't likely to cause harm, ingestion of prior to the event can create a negative feeling. In the end, the moment it happens the topic, you'll become aware of how harmful alcohol can be not just within your bowels, but across the entire body.

My experience has been that the faster I consume alcohol following an Ayahuasca ceremony, the less the time that the glow of the ayahuasca ceremony is.

Weed and Ayahuasca

Traditional dieta also advises users to avoid any other prescriptions and drugs prior to taking Madre. But, there are religious groups or shamans, as well as organizations which make use of large quantities of both ayahuasca and cannabis and ayahuasca, often together. This method is controversial. debate.

I suggest you experiment using different situations. Participate in an ayahuasca-based ceremony, and abstain from marijuana. This can assist in gaining an understanding of the power of this plant's spirit.

Experience an Santa Maria Daime performance in the sanctification of marijuana in the concentraco, and huge portions of fats are passed around the rows, with every person performing the gesture of the cross, before smoking a huge inhale till all the church has been heated.

Ayahuasca as well as coffee

Dieta requires the avoidance of all kinds of stimulation - physical, social physical, emotional, or and culinary... Coffee has the ability to interfere with your detox and consuming coffee prior to ceremonies could cause the elimination very painful.

The majority of shamans suggest you avoid drinking caffeine or coffee throughout the course of your diet, and you should wean yourself off coffee prior to starting the dieta, if you do use regularly.

What To Avoid Prior Ayahuasca Diet

Eliminating Sugars, including artificial Sugars, prior to taking Ayahuasca (natural sugars that are found in maple syrup, honey and fruits are safe)

The red meat (Chicken and fish fine)

Pork

Vegetable Oils vs. Animal Fats

Culturally-inspired foods

Dairy Products (Eggs OK)

Caffeine (black coffee, or black tea that is not milked is okay)

Herbs, spices and other herbs are aromatic.

What to Eat

Consume, raw or steaming vegetables

The Fabaceae family includes legumes as well as beans and peas.

Cereal grains such as rice, Oats, buckwheat and barley

Fruit drinks, healthy snacks as well as fresh fruit

Use olive oil or Ghee in place of other oils when cooking. Also, eliminate your fried foods for a healthier alternative.

Freshly laid organic eggs. Not in the event of a big celebration.

Prescription Drugs

Numerous facilities suggest that you avoid taking these medication in the days leading towards the wedding

Antidepressants SSRI type

MAO-inhibitors

The use of medication for sleeping

Barbiturates

Beta-blockers and contraceptives

Dangerous Substances Found on the Streets

Amphetamines, cocaine, opiates marijuana, marijuana, and the drug methylphenidate (MDMA) are just a few instances. Also, it is recommended to avoid other psychedelics, such as LSD and psilocybin.

The women who are taking birth control pills may also discontinue taking them five days prior to their visit and the entire period they're there.

THE POST-AYAHUASCA DIET

What To Avoid

The next three days, be sure to ensure that you keep your head away from the direct sun and away from the water.

Avoid spicy meals for the next two weeks.

Alcohol or drugs that facilitate sexual activities

Frosty drinks and icy treats

The consumption of cannabis, pork and other herbal medicines must be kept away for two or four weeks following the treatment.

Massage and energy therapy are illegal drugs (cocaine, LSD, MDMA amphetamines, and so on.) To Eat

What To Eat

Fruits and vegetables that are edible (except citrus and overly acidic fruit in the initial 14 days)

Do not eat more than two portions of fruits each day during the first five days.

The teas made from plants like peppermint and the chamomile tea, do not contain caffeine.

If you are planning to consume an alternative to coffee for your drink, like a barley-based drink or dandelion root make sure you check the label to confirm that all the ingredients are natural and sugar-free.

Amaranth, rice, quinoa along with buckwheat, amaranth, quinoa, and other cereal grains

Beans, peas as well as other legumes (beans and chickpeas following 5 days)

Onions as well as garlic, ginger along with other fresh herbs, spice

Spices like cinnamon, nutmeg and cloves and allspice

Seedlings and cereals that have germinated

Olive oil or coconut that is five days old

We suggest that you avoid gluten for at least five days when you eat Oats Bread.

The pasta dishes are a good example, as is the pasta as well as rice-based (check ingredients lists to find the ingredients that contain preservatives)

The ideal chicken is free-range and organic.

Unconfined eggs from hens, best organic

Seafood (avoid the salmon or any other fat fish during the first five days) (avoid salmon or any other oilsy fish during the initial five days)

After five days, only some nuts can be consumed.

In the next 5 days, some pieces of dried fruit are enough.

Foods greatly benefit by the addition of grounded and soaked seeds like flaxseed, chia and sunflower or pumpkin.

Following day 5, just some honey is required (1 teaspoon at one period of)

After five days, Spirulina, Maca, and Cacao can be consumed safely.

Pea After the 5th day of the program it is safe to make use of protein powders to build the muscle.

At the end of day 5 you can consume non-dairy milk such as almond, soy or coconut milk. However, ensure there's no preservatives or sugar added.

Chapter 13: Why Are Diet And Preparation So Important?

It is essential to understand that your body functions as an instrument in the context of ayahuasca's use as a medicinal. The healthier and more fit that you're in, better you'll be able to be able to accept the ayahuasca medication. It is common knowledge to lead a healthier life as we get older, but the months leading towards getting to Pachamama are the best moment to begin. This means that the physical vessel you are in will possess an energetic boost and it will be at fully able to take in the benefits of plant medicines. The strictest adherence to these requirements will enable ayahuasca's function to be better and offer you an experience that is beneficial.

Dietas prepare the body for the consumption of ayahuasca, in the same manner as yoga poses are designed to prepare your body for a meditation as yoga.

In the present day our bodies gather huge amounts of information through our bodies.

Ideas, emotions and even external stimulations each leave a mark upon our body. When your body gathers and filters the information that is a part of your environment, you could be blocked or 'clogged.' These physical impressions can have significant implications for your health as well as the daily routine.

The most remarkable features of herbal remedies is the fact that they are able in restoring flow through the body, eliminating blocks and allowing the flow of life and energy to go more easily. The plant remedies can help people who are dieting to feel completely refreshed and reset so that they can move forward more easily without physical and mental restrictions which previously held their behind.

An intense diet during the weeks prior to, during and after your retreat is a must; it isn't easy to turn down the delicious food you eat. If you do this you'll show your dedication and commitment towards healing, as well as lay the basis for healing the body, mind, as well as the spirit.

Keep in mind that if the diet is viewed as an examination of willpower it's simple to comprehend that the exercise of abstaining from food and drink only scratches the top of the iceberg. Feeling dissatisfied, complaining about your diet, pondering about sexual desire, or lusting for certain foods are signs of determination, or absence of it.

Be careful not to be upset, doubting or losing faith when you are in the middle Thinking negatively regarding Dieta are important considerations. Dieta is not just about food. Dieta doesn't stop at food items.

It happens all day, and even during sleep.

Also, during the time afterwards, you should be sure to treat your body with respect and consideration. Every serious participant is required to stick to the recommended food restrictions.

AYAHUASCA DIET RECIPES

Gently Spiced Pumpkin Soup

Sautee Add one large onion chopped, and three garlic cloves (with or without oil) (simply make use of a small amount of water if at the beginning of 5 days)

Toss in 1 Tbsp. of fresh grated ginger, and 1 TBSP. of ground of cumin.

2.25 cups pumpkin or butternut squash cut in half and removed from the skin.

Add one cup sweet potato, by chop it.

Boil everything until the food is cooked to your liking.

Blender or hand blender to blend until it is smooth.

Salt and pepper according to your taste. Finally, top with fresh chopped coriander leaves and serve it in a beautiful way.

(after the 5th day, after day 5, you could add organic coconut milk as well as some or all ginger depending on your the taste).

A Lentil Bolognese

In a pot prepare the onions and garlic until cooked through.

Make 2 cups of lentils in brown and then add them to the pot.

It's equivalent to 2 cups of tomatoes that are fresh, cut into dices

Include one teaspoon of dried oregano, or Italian seasonings.

1 cup of water

1 tbsp. of tomato paste (check for any preservatives)

Add salt and pepper after the mixture has thickened and become an Bolognese sauce.

Begin your spaghetti meal with freshly chopped basil.

Roast Veg Salad

Sweet potatoes beets and pumpkins and carrots are great for this recipe, however it is also possible to use alternatives like zucchini and bell peppers. Roast the vegetables in the oven till they are brown and soft by throwing them into a little quantity of olive oil as well as salt. In order to prevent them becoming dry if you do not apply oil, add a little water onto the tray and protect it with aluminum foil.

Mix cooked roasted vegetables in the salad you like best of mixed greens. There is also the option of putting eggs that have been hardboiled over it should you wish to. Serve with avocado slices in the event that it's been longer than five days since you last had it, and roasting pumpkin seeds and sunflower seeds. Sprinkle some fresh, green herbs like basil or parsley. Add it with pepper and salt.

Banana Cakes

[[

Two bananas mashed should be mixed into one bowl.

Include 2 tablespoons. of Chia seeds.

1 egg (leave out this for the vegan option) (leave the egg out to make vegan alternatives)

Mix in 1/2 cup flour that is gluten-free, if you are using it, and one teaspoon of salt.

Turn the batter to the other side and give it a vigorous stir. You can add any additional water needed for the batter to reach an ideal pancake consistency. If you've got some blueberries, toss them into the batter as well.

The best option is to cook in the nonstick cooking pan, or even a tiny amounts of coconut oil during making.

Sprinkle fresh fruit on top and serve.

Breakfast oats!

1 cup rolled oatmeal

Include 2 tablespoons. of Chia seeds.

One tablespoon's worth

1 teaspoon ground cinnamon

1. Tsp. honey

One cup of water.

Place everything in a pot and heat on low with the addition of water if needed. On Day 5, you are able to utilize nut milks like almond milk or soymilk However, be sure there isn't any extra sugar or preservatives. Take it with a fruit that is that are fresh like papaya, a banana or a bowl full of fruit. For better digestion, crushing all of seeds prior to adding to the oatmeal is an excellent idea.

Full-Power Anti-Flam Chicken Broth

The easiest method to use is to utilize an electric slow cooker. If you feel tired after eating the food that is medicinal can be an excellent option for increasing your endurance and helping improve digestion health. Put a whole organic free-range chicken in the slow cooker, and then fill all the remaining space with water.

Blend in 1 teaspoon of finely grated fresh ginger. Mix in one teaspoon fresh grated turmeric a peeled and mashed clove of garlic a pinch on black pepper a quarter one teaspoon of salt as well as a pinch of salt.

Set it to low and allow it to simmer through the through the night.

The chicken should be removed out of the soup along with bones at the beginning of the day. The chicken's carcass can be enjoyed as is or shred and added to the soup, creating the most delicious stew of chicken vegetables.

Place the bones back in the soup and cook for an additional 3 hours on low.

Bones, everything else Pour the broth into an strainer before throwing it away.

When the soup is settled and the soup is cooled, you can remove any fat that's left by skimming it off of the surface. If you're not feeling weak or overweight, it's best to retain the soup.

Once the soup has cool and the broth is cool, you are able to keep it in the refrigerator for about a week, or store it in the freezer to use later. Make it into the sauce that you use to cook vegetables as well as to cook grain such as quinoa or rice. For healing the digestive tract that has been damaged and boost the strength of your immune system, take this soup. It is high in minerals, collagen and anti-inflammatory benefits.

AN OVERVIEW OF THE AYAHUASCA DIET'S EFFECTS

The Mental Effects of Ayahuasca

The various regions of the right hemisphere brain, as per the latest research, are more active as a result of use. In addition, these brain regions are linked to emotional self-awareness and processing of feelings and different aspects of emotion-related cognition.

It is therefore dangerous to mix ayahuasca and the class of antidepressants referred to as selective serotonin Reuptake Inhibitors. Serotonin in huge quantities are created by this combination. In the event of the "overdose" of serotonin in the brain, there is serotonin syndrome.

Signs and symptoms include symptoms like cold sweats, diarrhea elevated body temperature, as well as irregular heartbeats. The airways become constricted and respiratory problems, and finally the death of a patient can occur.

Psychological Effects

Mind-body effects that have been associated with the use of ayahuasca can be described as:

The process of dissociating oneself from his personal thoughts and emotions is called depersonalization.

Alterations in spatial and temporal perception, as well as impaired proprioception and body awareness.

Hallucinations both visual and auditory. visual

Astral projection

The feeling of saturated colors

The lack of authority

In a state of confusion, bewilderment

Positive emotions that promote positivity

On the other hand, it is possible to feel negative emotions like anxiety, sadness, anger or even a sense of agitation.

The fear of losing one's mind or life

Unsettling or disturbing images or sound

Memories of sad or traumatic events memories

experiences of revelations, typically that are of an extraterrestrial or spiritual kind.

Physiological Side Effects

Most commonly, the negative side effects include nausea, and frequently vomiting. A few people who take the medicine also experience diarrhoea. This is considered to be positive in the shamanic worldview as they show that the medication is performing its job by flushing out toxic substances from the body, mind and even the spirit.

Other impacts are:

Being diagnosed with an abnormally high blood pressure

Acceleration of the Heartbeat

Seizures

Tremors

Pupillary dilation

Involuntary, rapid, continuous eye movement is known as nystagmus.

Dizziness

Incoordination is often referred to as ataxia

A feeling of nausea and nausea and vomiting (typically when consumed orally the ayahuasca)

Chapter 14: Possibility Of Developing Psychosis

Flashbacks that are recurrent, psychological, and hallucinations are just a few of the adverse results of long-term consumption. The effects of these side effects might be present for months,, or perhaps years later after the end of the use of this drug.

Persistent psychosis, a term used in medicine, is the name for the disorder. In addition, those who have mental illness tend to suffer from this. But the truth is that everyone can suffer from this even after just one attempt at a psychedelic.

They are just a few indicators of long-term psychosis

Mental illnesses

Brain cluttered

The fear that will not be able to

Eye irritation.

Hallucinogen-Induced Persistent Perception Disorder

Another mental health issue linked to heavy psychedelic usage is hallucinogen-persisting perception disorder (HPPD). Additionally people who struggle with mental health issues are more affected.

The signs that indicate HPPD can be seen as follows:

Hallucinations

Another visual distortion include following the movement of objects with your eyes, or spotting halos on stationery objects

signs that can be identical to symptoms of neurologic illness, like a stroke brain tumor.

MEDICAL GUIDELINES ASSOCIATED WITH AYAHAUSCA DIET

The healing methods we practice are based in the shamanic practice of ancient times of medicinal plants from the Amazon. Ayahuasca, as well as other medicinal plants that we use are extremely powerful biochemically and energetically however, they do not always go together with other medications.

A few physical or psychological conditions cannot be treated using ayahuasca. Likewise, the usage of many prescription medications, natural supplements as well as plants, isn't secure when used in conjunction with this drug.

Talk to us prior to abstaining completely If you're not able to drink ayahuasca as it is possible that there are other alternatives that can be used in place.

Guests must discuss the safe withdrawal of their medications with their physician and us in accordance with the guidelines of The Garden of Peace. In the moment of submitting an applying for an event or retreat, any medical preexisting or current concerns must be reported.

The ailments, medicines and other supplements mentioned below are just a small selection of the numerous that must be avoided when taking Ayahuasca. If you have a health issue that is not listed, contact us as well as your physician.

Because heart-related irregularities may not be detected until the test is conducted, we recommend everyone who visits us to take a full medical exam prior to working with us. We will recommend a certified physician in the region that you're currently in.

In the case of illnesses for which Ayahuasca isn't the appropriate treatment

Schizophrenia

manic-depressive illness

Suicidal thoughts, antisocial behavior and depression are other examples of dissociative diseases.

Severe cardiac problems

The usage of Ayahuasca shouldn't be mixed with any other medication or other supplements. Unless specifically stated, visitors aren't allowed to take any medication or nutritional supplements throughout their stay. It's essential to quit specific drugs for at least one month before beginning to use Ayahuasca or a different Master Plant. Talk to our team and with your physician in order to figure out the time it'll take to allow a specific substance be eliminated from your body and the impacts, if any that you could experience once you begin working with our company.

These drugs are not recommended to be taken while taking Ayahuasca.

SSRIs (any specific serotonin Reuptake Inhibitor) (any Serotonin selective Reuptake Inhibitor)

amphetamines (meth-, dex-, amphetamine) (meth-, dex-, amphetamine)

Antihypertensives (high blood pressure medicine) (high blood pressure medication) appetite suppressants (diet medications) (diet pills)

Treatments for respiratory conditions

treatment for colds, allergies as well as sinus conditions (Actifed DM, Benadryl, Benylin Chlor-Trimeton Compiz and more.)

The medications that can slow down the nervous system's central part

antipsychotics

alcohol

The herbs do not interact with diet supplements.

Herb of St. John

Kava

Ephedra

Ginseng

YohimbeSinicuichi

Certain medicines shouldn't be taken with Ayahuasca.

Actifed

Amantadine Hydrochloride

Amoxapine (Asendin)

Benadryl

Benylin

Bupropion (Wellbutrin)

Buspirone (BuSpar)

Carbamazepine (Tegretol, Epitol)

Chlor-Trimeton

Clomipramine (Anafranil)

Cocaine

Cyclobenzaprine (Flexeril)

Cyclizine (Marezine)

Desipramine (Pertofrane)

Dextromethorphan (DXM)

Disopyramide (Norpace)

Doxepin (Sinequan)

Ephedrine

Hydrochloride Flavoxate (Urispas)

Fluoxetine (Prozac)

Imipramine (Tofranil)

Isocarboxazid (Marplan)

Levodopa (Dopar, Larodopa

Loratadine (Claritin) (Claritin)

Maprotiline (Ludiomil) (Ludiomil)

Meperidine (Demerol)

Methylphenidate (Ritalin)

Nortriptyline (Aventyl)

Chlorobutynol oxidase inhibitor (Ditropan)

Orphenadrine (Norflex)

Parnate

Paroxetine (Paxil)

Phenergan

Phenelzine (Nardil)

Procainamide (Pronestyl)

Protriptyline (Vivactil)

Pseudoephedrine

Quinidine (Quinidex)

Salbutamol

Salmeterol

Selegiline (Eldepryl)

Sertraline (Zoloft)

Tegretol

Temaril

Tranylcypromine (Parnate)

Treatment of depression by tricyclic antidepressants (Amitriptyline, Elavil)

Trimipramine (Surmontil)

Yohimbine

BENEFITS OF THE AYAHAUSCA DIET

Many mental, physical as well as spiritual issues were treated by Ayahuasca. It is an effective method for healing and personal growth, cleansing, and a greater understanding.

At times, participants experience a deep spiritual connection as well as a greater understanding of their own lives, self and the very nature of existence. The medicine, when used with other master plant species makes a potent tool that can treat a myriad of ailments that impact the body, mind and the soul.

Check out our Healing Tales page to learn the stories of our fellow guests, and do not hesitate to get in touch with us if you have questions.

Each ritual is different; simply accepting whatever happens trusting in the process and spending the time to reflect on the experience afterwards can assist you in getting maximum benefit from the Ayahuasca ceremonies. Ayahuasca affects the most profound cell levels of illness emotional, energy, and mood that require the time needed to integrate properly.

Chapter 15: What Is Ayahuasca?

The History of Ayahuasca

There are many indigenous groups that reside in South America that use the Ayahuasca vine as an effective treatment for ailments and for facilitating treatment and heals. As there aren't documents that document when the practice first began however, it's hard to determine exactly the length of time Ayahuasca was used by Shamans to treat ailments as a healer. But, there are oral records of an indigenous people's recipe for an ayahuasca-brewed brew that was developed around 5,000 years ago.

Spanish as well as Portuguese missionaries arrived in South America during the 16th century and became acquainted with ayahuasca, ayahuasca used by indigenous South Americans. With their narrow-minded view belief, the healing power of the plant was Devil's work. It also sparked debate regarding its usage between diverse beliefs and cultures. They didn't inquire into the curative properties of ayahuasca and as a result, Ayahuasca was largely unknown beyond the Amazon region up until the beginning of the 20th century.

In 1908, researchers in the West recognized the existence of Ayahuasca, as well as its mystical properties. This is attributed the work of Richard Spruce, a British botanist who traveled in South America to classify the tea's components. He also wrote about benefits of the purging effect of medicines and the importance of this concoction made from a master plant in the history and lifestyle of the Amazonian people.

The practice of purification is a religion and a popular belief that it is a way to let go of any negativity that's blocked energy from properly flow through your subtle body, as well as your physical body. The process is carried out using a variety of techniques, but the most popular is vomiting and diarrhea. Ayahuasca is also believed designed to cleanse the body of parasites and the worms.

Shamans believe that Shamans are of the opinion that negative energies cause diseases and illness. They believe that it ought to be considered a positive element rather than an unpleasant alternative.

The interest in the healing and spiritual properties of ayahuasca at its peak in the 1960s as the works were composed by Richard Evans Schultes and brothers Dennis & Terance McKenna. The books were called The Yage Letters and True Hallucinations in the respective books. They narrated their own experiences with the drink of ayahuasca within the Amazon. Even in the midst of hippie movement and the psychedelic revival that was taking place at the time, interest in the healing plant did been largely ignored as one were still required to make trips to the Amazon jungle at that moment.

Master plants are among the most effective teachers in the world of nature. They have the ability to connect with people with whom they have had long-lasting friendship with them for an extended period of time. They can establish trust and respect with the plant as well as the essence of the plant. They are also receiving information about the benefits of the plant, and possibly other plants that can help in achieving the ultimate purpose. The Shamans are known as doctores, which is the Spanish term for doctor since they play as if they were.

The tale of Schultes has inspired the journalist William S. Burroughs to visit the Amazon to find the cure or cure for addiction to opiate. The psychologist Claudio Narajo by making the trek through the Amazon River in a canoe at the beginning of 1970. Narajo was a scientist who studied ayahuasca alongside the South American Indians and then afterward released The Healing Journey which included his research on the alkaloids that are active in the plant's master, which was the first one of its kind.

The most prominent proponent of the benefits of ayahuasca, is an English journalist from Britain known as Graham Hancock. The journalist is candid about how the psychedelics affect our consciousness and how humans share long-standing connections to these master healing plants. He also candidly discusses his own experiences with a variety of forms of psychedelic drugs across the world. He was also included in a TED Talk. But his talk The War on Consciousness was disqualified for his conversation about how these substances change our perception with a profound way.

Ayahuasca is extensively used in healing and medical purposes throughout the ages. According to research, the Shamans from Peru have shared their knowledge of the plant's mastery with those of the Mestizo holy people, who spread the knowledge of caring for patients in the Amazon. There are Amazonian indigenous people who use the ayahuasca plant for healing and insights primarily in the jungles that are Brazil, Ecuador, Colombia and Peru.

In the present, ayahuasca is a unique ingredient in Brazil because it is integrated into the Christian religion. The religious movement of Uniao do Vegetal and Santo Daime are also gaining the acclaim of their followers and are now used to create churches across the world. They only use the original blend of master plants. They do not mix any other admixtures with the drink during ceremonies.

Quechua is the name of the native language used in the majority of the Amazon Basin. It's derived composed of two words that are from the spoken language that ayahuasca was coined to refer to the vine. "Aya" means dead or soul "Huasca" is defined as the rope, or woody vine. Therefore, the literal translation of Ayahuasca is Vine of the Spirits Vine of the Dead, or Vine of the Souls.

Another meaning of Ayahuasca is The Rope of the Spirits. It is because of the connection that this plant symbolizes between the spiritual world and the physical world that we inhabit everyday.

The Growing Popularity of Aya

Prior to the time when drinking this sacred drink became widely known, it was necessary travel to far-off regions in South America to participate. In response to the overwhelming demand of Westerners to experience this mystical moment, there were many retreat facilities created to serve precisely this reason. The spread of information about ayahuasca has proven to be extremely effective and centers are opening all across the world. These retreats offer the luxury and comforts that are not available in traditional ceremonies that were held in the midst that are part of the Amazon. But, it also opened an opportunity to many who didn't want to explore new territories by themselves and provided a means for Westerners to take advantage of this healing in a protected location.

In light of the growing understanding of Ayahuasca and its benefits, it can be located in many places across the world. There is an interest among Westerners who have been taken to the jungles that are South America with Shamans to study the practice and to establish an ongoing relationship with Ayahuasca as well as other plants that teach.

They're following the same method of initiation that many Shamans had learned prior to they by working with a variety of master plant educators as well as ayahuasca to learn about the healing powers of these plants. It is also an essential step which aids in spreading Ayahuasca's healing all over the globe since this group of Western participants will be able to lead ceremonies using ayahuasca either at home in their countries of origin or at the retreat centers.

The Amazonian practices differ greatly from what is commonly a Western viewpoint that it is necessary to be aware of the different values that the Amazonian people hold.

Because they are in a constant relationship with the Earth and with co-habitants and the earth, they don't hold to the material objects that exist in this world. They can gain an insightful outlook on death as well as the best way to live their lives as fully as feasible outside of themselves.

If you're participating in an Ayahuasca-based ceremony you must be aware that this is just an act of a small magnitude that Amazonian peoples shamans carry out in the larger picture in their daily lives.

Chapter 16: The Science Of Ayahuasca

The Components of Ayahuasca

The ayahuasca vine consists of the tetrahydroharmine (THH) harmaline, tetrahydroharmine (THH), as well as harmine alkaloids. The THH alkaloids constitute an insignificant type of serotonin Reuptake Inhibitor (SRI). THH plays a role in inhibiting the absorption of serotonin in the presynaptic neuron as well as platelets.

Alkaloids harmine and harmaline are MAOI elements that are responsible for stimulating your central nervous system. Alkaloids are also responsible in ensuring that Dimethyltryptamine which is more often referred to as DMT and isn't metabolized through the acidic environment of stomachs, allowing the drug to be processed by the liver. Once DMT is able to cross the blood brain barrier, the emotional epiphanies can last for a long time and form the base for the effects of purging that you may feel.

How Ayahuasca Affects the Brain

The harmine alkaloids and harmine can be beneficial to the brain because they increase the production of dopamine that acts as an antidepressant. It also improves individuals' mood. Additionally, they reduce withdrawal symptoms that are associated with recreational and painkillers. substances.

They also increase levels of brain-derived neurotrophic factors (BDNF) found within the hippocampus area within the cortex. The BDNF is the main reason for long-term memory as well for the growth of neurons.

A well-known study which was carried out on participants of the UDV church that concluded that those who had been long-term people who took ayahuasca experienced more than the normal amount 5HT-related brain transporters. In the past, although there wasn't any research on elevated levels of 5HT, but they were referring to studies with very low levels of those same transporters.

If you have a loved one who has lower levels of 5HT are typically afflicted with the urge to eat, suicidal thinking violence, and alcoholism. Researchers have determined this due to the levels of THH that are present in the Aya beer.

The MAOIs can also be responsible to reduce cravings as well can be helpful for addiction issues which may occur due to the dopaminergic systems.

How Shamans Work the Ayahuasca Vine

Madre Ayahuasca is considered to be the mother spirit of the jungle and has the power to govern all other spirits in the jungle.

The indigenous people from the Amazon have been working so closely with the plants of sacred significance for many years following their first initiation They are able to identify the many varieties of the ayahuasca grapevine. They don't adhere to the Westernized method of taxonomy since they are aware that it wouldn't be accurate to categorize them in that way.

It is because of their understanding of different strains with diverse healing properties based upon the kind of visions they cause, the spiritual significance of the place they are located and the date they have to be harvested, as and the kind of soil they grow. It is also possible to identify them based on the colors of visions they trigger like black, yellow blue, white and red.

Other species are named after species that can be observed, such as boa, jaguar, and monkey. The master plants can be seen because they communicate by a variety of senses, as well and through non-sensory methods. Since shamans have close connections with spirits, they have the ability to perceive every way they can communicate.

It's hard to some people to believe that the Amazonian indigenous peoples have recorded around 80 percent of the native species of plants found within the rainforest. It's a tiny percentage in comparison to the one-million additional to be catalogued. But, having identified this vast quantity of plants and are aware of an understanding about the properties that heal every one, but it is difficult to ask the way they managed to attain this vast quantity of knowledge within a relatively very short time.

It is believed that the South American Indian explain that they believed that it was Madre Ayahuasca communicating through the vine, guiding and educate them about the qualities of other plant species that were needed to heal. Because of this intimate connection to the vine skilled Shamans could discern the type of vine at a reasonable distance, and could speak to Spirit. Spirit without having to ingest the plant.

A person who has a logical brain would find the process that is based on trial and error as not be very effective with regard to the vast number of plants that heal.

In the traditional world, it's commonly used by shamans and healers to facilitate the connection with nature. Spiritual leaders may also employ it to discover what's causing people to get sick at the level of spirituality.

Shamans utilize ayahuasca for healing all over to communicate with the energies that nature has to offer and treat psychological traumas. Through communication to nature's Spirit of Vine the Shaman seeks to acquire the expertise to treat and heal diseases. It also assisted them in different community issues. Additionally, they would utilize the data provided to them by Spirit of the plant Spirit from the plants to identify the person's love for their spouse. They also would use this information to implement rituals that were black magic to people in the group.

Before it became popular in the past, Shaman was the Shaman was the only one who could participate in the ritual for guidance on the best way to heal individuals physically and spiritually by the spirit of plants. In the past, people in the community would consume the mixture only at least once in their lives. The reason for this was extreme and painful circumstances that could arise as well as the respect they had for the Shaman who was in numerous relationships and with his Master

Plant to perform the cleansing work. This ceremony has changed due to the surge of curiosity about this Vine of the Soul.

In order to develop a connection with the plant that is Master of all To develop a relationship with this plant, the Shamans were required to spend a long period of time, sometimes stretching up to five years in order to eat and interact in The Spirit of the Vine as along with other plants used as teachers in order to understand their benefits as well as their effects. The journeys to these plants formed part of the regimented diet that had to be adhered to. It helped them make use of the information obtained to improve the lives of those who live there, as well as the surrounding surroundings and community overall through being able to inquire questions to the Mother Spirit who guided them through their studies.

In this phase of initiation, the student creates the pharmacy of plants that can manage a wide range of diseases to the people in their group. The students spend a lot of time in each tree and master plant they're instructed to utilize via Madre Ayahuasca which is can be a very taxing task as the student is pushed towards the edges of their physical, mental and spiritual capacities. They are incredibly strong and the power which is felt when you have a full connection with their energy is enormous as ayahuasca is not the most powerful among the master plants. The Shamans will gain a greater understanding and appreciation of the Shamans when you experience ayahuasca's potent energy.

Also, they adhere to the strict diet advised to all participants of the ceremony in order to attain all the knowledge Mother Ayahuasca yearns to give. This diet is free of sugar, oil, and unripe, baked bananas along with white rice. It is in addition to the master plant's drinks. The type of diet initiated by an initiate through taking cleansing emetics, such as yawarpanga and sacred tobacco. If they are performing the purgatory rituals in similar reasons that Shamans are likely to suggest following an identical diet prior to your ceremony. It puts the initiate's body in a condition that permits the plant to provide maximum beneficial effects.

The Science of Ayahuasca Tea

The brewing process can take anywhere from 8 hours to just a couple of days, based upon the recipe. The basic brewing preparation involve cultivating the Banisteriopsis caapi plant cutting approximately two meters of the plant in order to create one batch of tea. The leaves, branches and the bark are taken away and broken into smaller segments. The pulp is crushed until it is small fibres.

In the morning, when the brew has ready to be prepared, leafy chacruna leaves plant are collected and mixed with dried leaves in a boiling pot of fifty liters. The pot is filled with approximately 40 Liters of water in the pot to cover the master plant and let the mix slow boil for approximately 8 hours. The plant matter is removed by straining it through a sieve. About 1 liters of the ayahuasca tea is left. The amount of tea consumed per person is around 2 to 3 pounds.

You must take great care when you prepare this recipe as you could overcook your brew, and destroy the therapeutic characteristics of the beverage. It is a method of science people of indigenous origin hold to be cherished. The tourism industry is growing rapidly and growing, you will discover ayahuasca virtually everywhere on the road, even at markets selling it in basic soda bottles. The roadside vendors lure the unsuspecting tourists to purchase the fake brew at around 100 dollars, and they have no information about the person who made the drink, or what it is made of, or if it's genuine.

It's made up of an amalgamation of the Ayahuasca plant, scientifically referred to as Banisteriopsis caapi, and Psychotria viridis leaves, which are known under the term chacruna, which is a translation of mix. Additionally, there are medicinal plants which certain tribes include to the mix, such as

Brugmansia, toe, and produce different effects on the person who is taking part. There's a certain procedure that the Shamans make the drink and the whole procedure revolves around rituals, singing, and the creation of environment to allow to allow the Spirit mother of the vine along with her fellow plant spirits masters to work together.

The entheogenic nature of the drink of ayahuasca has diverse names, based upon the region of South America you are partaking. The plant used to teach is known by many names, including the purga, yage, la medicina Aya caapi, caapi and daime just to name some.

DMT is the principal ingredient in the chacruna plant that is the reason for the psychedelic experience when you drink the tea that is brewed in Ayahuasca. DMT can be found naturally in brains of animals as well as in the plants itself naturally. It is a serotonin-based neurotransmitter and interacts in conjunction with neural circuits, primarily within the frontal cortex the amygdala and hippocampus.

The location of where the plants are harvested, and the period of the year it is, amount of alkaloid will vary. Additionally, the beverage contains a higher quantity of alkaloids than plants. The average amount of 200ml would be around 25 mg of DMT 10 mg THH, and thirty mg harmine/harmaline.

It is thought it is believed that Psychotria viridis was added to produce a more concentrated empiric to assist in the removal of parasites that are present in our bodies. The study found that when the two plants were combined that the visual aspect was greatly affected, more so than making use of the ayahuasca tree by itself.

The belief is that the mixture of chacruna was conceived after the awe-inspiring beneficial effects of ayahuasca began to spread throughout all over the world. According to all reports this is a brand new evolution in the long-standing time of indigenous Amazonian peoples, who exclusively made use of the ayahuasca grapevine to aid in divination rituals and treatment.

How Ayahuasca Tea Affects the Brain

If these regions that are influenced due to serotonin levels that are disrupted by the 5-HT2A receptors the effects are profound of the introspection and emotional processing. The same receptors that get active in other psychedelics including psilocybin, a.k.a LSD. As DMT is a brain chemical similarly to SSRIs and SSRIs, the mood increases. The brain regions which are impacted by DMT are the frontal cortex and pineal gland as well as the amygdala, and hippocampus.

The frontal lobe of the brain is the brain region which is accountable for a variety of diverse aspects of consciousness. For instance, it is which is where memories are stored. emotions of empathy, and the ability to communicate. The pineal gland becomes active as your physical body remains in a state of vulnerability that causes an expansion of consciousness. This leads to the search for our innermost self.

The hippocampus is that stores your emotional memories and it is part of your limbic system. It is also the place where memory that is long-term kept. The amygdala, too, is an area in the limbic system which is where the fear of one's self are built, as well as emotional memories and responses.

These areas of our brain energized this is that the benefits of drinking this beverage is based on memories and feelings associated to these experiences.

The study also found that the ayahuasca drink significantly decreased the occurrence of the default Mode Network (DMN) of the brain. The role for the DMN is to control how our brain interacts with its surroundings. It is evident when people who have experienced trauma that have occurred in their lives, causing an inclination to certain things that occur in their personal interactions. When certain events trigger these defaults within the DMN this acts as a catalyst to form cycles and, if ignored, they may result in mental health problems.

Ayahuasca reveals the origins of our feelings and responses that accompany the traumatizing events It breaks the normal behavior of the DMN to allow new, healthy habits can be developed. It is possible to break the cycle of hold these events that have caused trauma over you.

Also, it has been established that the mechanism behind Ayahuasca can promote mindfulness and disengagement from negative thinking patterns. The result is that participants are free from prior traumas, and being able to tackle the stressful situations of life with a more positive attitude.

In the case of consuming ayahuasca solely it produces visions which are void of form and appear only in the form of black and white. The reason for this is because of DMT with chacruna in it that the vision display becomes significantly enhanced.

There is a definite belief that the traditional diet followed by indigenous shamans results in an increased sensitivity to DMT. A typical Western diet is known to destroy DMT compounds that naturally exist in the brain, due to the high levels of monoamine oxidase enzymes consumed by people who have aged and processed food.

Since the shamans have developed this particular sensitivity solely through the consumption of ayahuasca they have the ability to adjust their focus to the healing power of the vine in a direct way. Westerners do not have the ability to get the same advantages from the ayahuasca vine which is why they are able to combine Chacruna and other mixtures are mixed to allow these people to get an experience it is possible to recover their physical, mental as well as spiritually.

The adverse effects of DMT which is found in the ayahuasca grape include an increase in cardiovascular and blood pressure levels, dilation of pupils, dizziness and anxiety. If you consume large amounts of DMT then you are likely to have seizures. The psychological side effects are visions of hallucinations as well as altered perceptions of reality.

The Spiritual Effect of Ayahuasca Tea

The appeal of The Master Plant is that it can connect you to the higher self. It helps to give you the understanding and understanding that you need for you to get the direction needed for resolving the issues you face in your daily life.

Similar to everything that is related to spiritual lines, this is not an easy task and it is essential to have the proper intention and respect in order to gain a better knowledge.

The drinking of yage isn't something to be done at random because it could alter your lifestyle as you are accustomed to it. Many people who aren't seeking a new psychedelic experience to add to their collection are aware of this and enter into the ritual with a sense of reverence. Because Aya is known as "the most truthful mirror It is difficult to be hesitant about this choice. It is important to be certain that you're ready to look at yourself in that way as it tears your own ego to pieces, which can make it feel like you are not part of the larger perspective of the Universe but ultimately, connected.

Ayahuasca will make one take a look at your beliefs of your ideologies, beliefs, and notions you use to define your self and personal identity. Ayahuasca reveals what you truly are and how that can help your future.

As the popularity of this brew it has been increased in certain instances in order to provide intense experiences for Western consumers. That's why people from indigenous groups can drink Aya several times in a month without experiencing a strong response to Aya. The reason is that they are using it in a different way and have an inferior mix, or even master plants alone.

In addition to the health issues which could arise The experience of taking Ayahuasca may not be suitable for all individual as it pushes your to the very limits of your capabilities from both sides of the scale. The casual consumer who is preparing on their first experience, they might hesitate to decide to this point. It is best to stay away from it since the vine must be revered for the purpose it serves as it's not a solution for any physical, mental or spiritual issue you may be suffering. While you may experience a an incredible experience that is unimaginable but you must make certain that the experience of connection with Mother Aya was worthwhile.

If you are feeling like you've lost your connection to the world around you, Shamanism may be the solution you are looking into. If we consider healers or Shamans They are in touch to both their personal and external realms through a profound knowledge of the energy that exist in both realms.

Utilizing plants for healing and to help is an integral part that people live their lives in their Amazon rainforest. They can also be your traveling companions while you strive to become a better version of you. When we travel this way The teacher plants help and help us to become your best friend. They want to remind you that life itself is holy and sacred.

The plants can heal due to their primary source of energy that comes from Mother Earth. The ability to embody the power of these plants in the event that the subtle and physical body energy is in order.

The Spirit's voice Spirit is feminine that is why she is known as Mother Spirit. Mother Spirit. The Spirit speaks via the plant of mastery in order to guide your attention to things that need to be addressed within your own life, to assist reaching your objectives.

If you're feeling that your heart is beckoning you to learn from Mother Aya chances are that she finds the way for you. Her intention is to plant a consciousness seed within your mind The path you take is bound to lead you to the point where you're ready to feel Her.

How Admixtures Affect the Tea

Some indigenous communities they use admixtures to mix different stimulants in the mix. This may not be the best choice for those who are first introduced to the drink. The reason is that the drinkers who are not tolerant with the indigenous population who drink regularly. Additionally, the intensity of these mixtures differs according to the season at which they harvest, which impacts the quantity of alkaloids in the.

It is important to be aware that there are additional admixtures in your tea which you may not be aware of are blended in with the tea. It is important to ask about the specific ingredients during the event you're going to so that you're fully aware of the substances you're infusing into your body. It could be that the ceremony takes a very different course with these ingredients. If the person you are facilitating is trustworthy and open about this details, there ought to not be any issues since they're the professionals and you should trust their advice.

There are a variety of popular admixtures used in the brewing of ayahuasca. They are used in conjunction with any other purging plant which are prescribed by specific Shamans to cleanse your body of any blockages. Make sure you ask your Shaman on the use of the plants, their benefits and potential side consequences to be informed of the potential side effects that could be felt during and after the ritual. Below is an overview of the ceremony.

* Remo Caspi bark (Aspidosperma excelsum) is a great remedy for dark and dense energy from the body's subtle energy. The main use for medicinal purposes is malaria. Other uses include cancer as well as diabetes,

inflammation Hepatitis, high blood pressure as well as digestive problems and fevers.

* Tamamuri (Brosimum Acutifolium) protects and helps to ward off energies which are ejected from individuals. Its medicinal benefits include the purification of blood, inflammation as well as fungal, parasite and arthritis. It also helps with cancer, Syphilis, and antibacterial.

* Chullachaki Caspi bark (Byrsonima Christianeae) is a plant that purifies which also assists in overcoming illnesses of the body.

*Capirona bark (Calycophyllum spruceanum) provides protection and cleansing. The medicinal uses of the bark include treating eye infections and fungal skin infections and it is also an anti-diabetic.

* Huacapurana (Campsiandra angustifolia) can be used to provide a grounding for the ceremony. The medicinal uses of this plant

include malaria, diarrhea, fever as well as Lyme's Disease.

* Wyra Caspi bark (Cedrelinga caeniformis) is a tranquilizer and helps to calm the mind. It also helps to rid the body of digestive and gastric disorders through eliminating.

* Lupuna Blanca bark (Ceiba pentandra) gives protection. Its medicinal benefits comprise Type II diabetes, headaches and diuretics.

* Ayahuma bark (Couroupita Guanensis) offers protection and healing to the soul which was abandoned due to spiritual trauma or fear. The medicinal uses of the bark include malaria, abdominal pain, inflammation swelling, hypertension and pain.

* Shiwawaku bark (Dipteryx odorata) offers the protection. Its medicinal benefits include the treatment of parasites and diarrhea.

* Camu camu Gigante (Myrciaria dubia) helps keep evil spirits and dark energy in check. The herb is used to treat cardiovascular diseases

as well as certain cancers, arthritis, and diabetes.

* Uchu Sanango (Tabernaemontana Sanaango) provides strength, power and security. In terms of medicine, it can be used to treat the treatment of pain and addiction to opiates. The primary alkaloid found in the plant is iboga, which is a psychoactive chemical that naturally exists. Iboga also has the same benefits of meditation and spiritual growth like ayahuasca.

* Punga Amarilla bark provides protection through the removal of negative energy from the subtle energy of your body.

Warns concerning Admixtures

Take care of the mixture of 5-MeO DMT which is also referred to by the term anadenanthera pilgrimage, yopo, or cohaba. The substance is known to be the cause of serotonin syndrome, and it interacts negatively with harmine and harmaline which can be found within harmine and harmaline, which are found in the ayahuasca vine. These effects are similar to what is found in ayahuasca vine. Shamans utilize yopo to boost the benefits of the tea. When it is mixed in the wrong way, negative side effects include permanent seizures, kidney damage high blood pressure, increased the temperature and heart rate as well as even, in the extreme even death.

The 5-MeO-DMT admixture is virolatheiodora, which is often referred to as red virola that also has DMT. It is used by South American Shamans as a Snort, and even more frighteningly in the form of poisoning of the arrow. The effects of this are hallucinations and lucid dreams. nightmare states, headaches and dizziness.

toe (Brugmansia) can be described as a hallucinogen that enhances the experience of vision due to the alkaloids in atropine and the scopolamine. Only a small portion of this mixture is enough because it's extremely potent, and provides a vibrant experience of

Mother Ayahuasca. However it could be dangerous when mixed improperly. Toe's side effects from an overdose can include seizures, a temporarily lost sight and dehydration. It can also cause poisoning seizures, pupils that are dilated as well as amnesia, hyperventilation hallucinations that resemble life as well as unconsciousness and possibly death in the extreme.

Also, be extremely cautious when mixing bufo alvarius that originates out of the Colorado River and Sonora Desert toad. It is a poisonous venom which is released from their skins and has begun to enter into tea ayahuasca. The side effects from an overdose of the ayahuasca admixture include permanently paralysis, seizures and deaths.

Chapter 17: Ayahuasca Ceremonies

Shaman or a Charlton?

Shamans are a group of people who Shamans are known by various names, based on the area in which they were born in. In the case of Amazonia, for instance, Shamans are known under their name Shipibo Ayahuasqueros, or Onanyas while Shamans from the Andes Mountains are known as Onanyas or Shipib Shamans who hail from in the Andean Mountains are referred to as Q'ero Paqos. The majority of indigenous people do not ever refer to them as Shamans because they are local physicians who guard and treat and are referred to generally as medical doctors.

In selecting the Shaman Begin a discussion with them before you make a decision. Stay off from any who has an online presence or comes directly to you offering the beverage. Shamans who are authentic to ayahuasca are silent and modest. It is possible to not be aware that they're Shamans at all because they're far from the spotlight. It is evident that real Shamans are affluent members of society. They live a happy existence and typically have an extended family. If they're isolated and mysterious, it could indicate that they might not want to be.

Over the course of their rigorous education, they've had to deal to their demons inside and out of Hell and then back. When they invite you to their sacred area of ceremony, they have agreed to guarantee that in the event you find yourself in a similar difficult situation they will be in the same place energetically in order to help you get out.

In all honesty, Shamans Shamans must be treated with the same respect that you show to the master plant itself.

If a healer begins their way to work alongside Madre Aya as well as being accepted as a student of shamanism. They are provided with a magical tool called darts referred to as the tsentsak. They are presented with these at introduction into the path, and are required to select either the dark or light path in which they will use them. They are exactly as they seem. They are able to penetrate the energy body's subtle energies and cause blockages which can cause illness, spiritual challenges and even death. Once the initiated Shaman is given the tsentsak, they're faced with the challenge of mastering their desire and use them to serve an higher cause and learns how to help others heal.

Since everyone has a choice but this doesn't mean that it is not the case for the religious Shamans since they are required to always choose to apply their powers of divination to benefit both the natural world and community. They may always choose to enter"the "dark aspect" creating witch doctors, or casting curses and spells too. Be careful and rely on your instincts in deciding who you're going to have to trust completely for the occasion.

There are those outside the indigenous groups and within them that are taking advantage of the chance to profit in sexual and ethical ways of innocent individuals. It is particularly true of locations where backpackers and tourists frequently look for the joy of awakening. These are the instances where ancient rituals may not be precise regarding what the first events were like in the isolated forests that are the Amazon and, more often than not, they're separated completely from the rituals that existed for a number of many thousands of years.

Be on the lookout for healers that clearly have mental issues or have addiction issues themselves, such as alcohol addiction. They also have pride in exaggerating about their abilities. There are criminals with no experience regarding the practices of shamanism and can cause hurt physically in order to obtain what they wish for. The so-called shamans might offer you what appears to be the ayahuasca drink, but they will not have it has no impact on the person you are. However the tea can cause the state of being in a state of obliviousness that could make you more susceptible.

This is why you should conduct your own research and make certain that you're being guided by a trained Shaman who has completed intense training in order to earn the designation. You must ensure you're working with a knowledgeable and dependable person capable of guiding you through the dark lands in which Ayahuasca might take you and explain different wonderful experiences are part of your experience so that you are able to get the most benefit of the information Mother Ayahuasca gives you to get the most out of your experiences.

There aren't so many well-trained Shamans than you imagine, since around 20 percent of all initiates get to the end of their path. It is evident that there are numerous individuals out there that have been through the process of studying the master plant. But, there's going to be more people who have only gained a little knowledge, however that is extremely risky when dealing with someone in the spiritual and energetic level that ayahuasca can provide. Of course, they'll know something about it to some extent and, as with studying the information contained in this book, it is not a way to make anyone an expert Shaman.

A lot of people conclude that the Shamans have been enlightened to the fullest extent. Certain may fit the Western standard. But the perspective and the belief system of Amazonian healers are very different from Western thinking because they have more in common with the natural world than we could ever be in the technological advancements of today's Western world. They have come to be accustomed to the diverse ecosystem in the Amazon and passed their principles down the generations, able to endure dangerous circumstances such as monsoon-like rains, dark spells from the sorcerers, vile entities toxic plants and creatures as well as illnesses.

The Shamans that you would like to collaborate with should have been in connection with Aya for minimum 10 years. That way, you are certain that they've been through many different situations and possess a solid understanding of the ayahuasca process. If you want to have a greater feeling of confidence in the Shaman's wisdom, ask about their family tree and whom they studied with. If they talk about the people mentioned, it must be done in a modest and respectful manner, without the appearance of boastfulness.

The real Shamans are people who transcend the desire to hurt others when they are in an impermanent state following the consumption of Ayahuasca tea. As they've gone through an intense course for healing through Mother Ayahuasca's healing power, they have acquired a tremendous commitment to never use the power of their channeling to do harm. If they're not capable of doing so it is because they are simply the sorcerer or witch doctor that lacks discipline and control over their behavior. It is more difficult than you think, as actually, the path that is darker and damaging people is a lot easier to follow than healing.

If you're working to a healer who is dark they could affect you in ways you're not aware of and can cause psychological and physical damage. In contrast to an authentic healer or Shaman and can trigger ailments in your body and the mind, and also make the power of demons and bad spirits. If a doctor chooses to take this route, it's mostly due to a absence of any experience in Spirit as well as the lack of the power of will that is required for the kind of work they're performing. This is precisely why that you should be vigilant in the process of determining which Shaman that you are dealing with and relying on at each level of your existence.

If an Shaman finds the right way of healing people and their surroundings They have a great degree of motivation to utilize their abilities to achieve the highest possible level of healing. If they keep following this route and continue to grow, they will be granted additional opportunities through the master plants and grow the healing abilities they channeled.

There are a myriad of Master Plants that can be used for healing previous traumas and emotional experiences psychological and spiritual ailments and energy imbalances. The understanding of Amazon Shaman traditions is that the Spirit of the Ayahuasca vine is the Mother of all Master plants. She also oversees the master plants below her. She can share along with the Shaman the incredibly healing wisdom that these plants possess. The Shaman becomes an intermediary to help work out to fulfill the wishes of the Master plants through healing patients.

Since the Amazonian existence is intertwined with the natural world and the spirit that reside in it, Shamans have a keen sense of imbalances in the world around them. They intuitively know the distinction between dense and light energies and are both malevolent as well as benevolent. They utilize this understanding to summon the various master plants necessary for the kind of ceremony being performed.

If you've discovered the right Shaman to collaborate with, make sure to talk with the Shaman as long as you can prior to making the choice to rely on his complete faith. Make use of your gut and contact the Shaman with all questions. They must be able to provide responses to all of your inquiries and should not evade the focus from the original questions. Shamans who are true Shamans are open, secure and seek to create an environment that is open and where everyone is at ease in the environment.

How Much Does a Ceremony Cost

There's a range of prices that come attending a wedding ceremony conducted by an individual Shaman who works independently as opposed to attending an all-inclusive retreat centre like you would anticipate. If you can locate an indigenous Shaman within your own community and communities, costs will be between $35 and 60 dollars for every ceremony you take part in. It is possible to stay in the community for one week is about $400. A breakfast and lunch is also included. Also, you'll enjoy the real experience of the Amazon when you stay within the tiny indigenous communities.

The cost of an retreat centre, you are intensive in terms of the preparation of and integration, it can cost between $800-$2000 to stay for the duration of a week. It includes food and being able to contact facilitators for all questions you might have and spa facilities including saunas, pools spas and massages. In addition, they usually provide extensive security in their facilities to make you are secure.

The Breakdown of the Ceremony

With the increasing popularization of Aya ceremony the fact is that the ceremony in itself is an entirely modernization in the history of South American Indian Shaman's practice. They have however used the mother

Vine for aid in providing directions for healing and also to aid in the practice of medicine.

The principal place that the indigenous tribes that perform ceremonies is located at the Amazon Basin in the northwest portion. Particularly, it is the place where Brazil, Ecuador, Peru and Columbia are joined. Additionally, there are communities of Mestizo communities which have an enviable presence within Pucallpa in Peru and Iquitos within Peru. You can also see the celebrations all over the world that are held in secret because DMT is classified as a Schedule I controlled substance, which is illegal without a specific religious purpose.

There are three kinds of ceremonies you can be involved in The traditional shaman ritual as well as the therapeutic or the ritual of religious significance.

Each ceremony will have Shaman, the facilitator, guiding the participants through the whole process prior to, during and following. The majority of ceremonies are conducted at the evening because there are fewer distractions of daily activities in the evening. There are occasions when the ceremony takes place in the morning. In bringing yourself into contact with the wisdom and master intelligence inherent in all human beings. It is likely that you will be connected to the source of everything you have ever known and will be on an adventure to places that which you could never imagine or even think of.

There are many individuals who have been certified to lead ceremonies. These include Padrinho, Therapist, healer or Mestre in the case of Ayahuasca ceremonies.

Ayahuasca sessions typically take place in groups of between five to twenty-five participants and occasionally, there could be more than 100 participants at a session, or even more.

Shaman is present to ensure that the Shaman is also in place to ensure order and harmony throughout the entire space. The Shaman is responsible for every person to ensure that the negative energy is dispersed with the help of spirit guides and enhance the energies of the area when needed by the Icarus. To make sure that the people are there, mobile phones as well as other electronic devices cannot be used within this sacred space since they could distract your fellow participants and you.

Deaths of those who have been reported as people who take Aya is directly due to their failure to follow the instructions from Shaman Shaman. It is also a matter of continuing to drink alcohol, drugs, and nicotine prior to the ceremony, as well as not being able to diagnose physical ailments. Many retreat facilities that insist on an up-to-date health screening for your protection at the time of your ceremony.

A designated shaman or facilitator will prepare ritually the tea ayahuasca on the day before the ceremony. Some retreat facilities also have others who create the medicine, and take it off to the location in addition. The amount of medicine depends on the group of professionals in the center.

Traditional Shaman Ceremony

The Shaman the neo-shaman or Vegetalistas are names used by the persons who conduct these ceremonies. They play an important element of the ritual since they have the responsibility of providing a secure space to allow the Ayahuasca Spirit as well as other spirits of the plant kingdom to perform their work, in healing your at a mental and emotional basis. The utmost confidence must be built up to the Shaman since you could be in the middle of some frightening or insightful experiences in which require an expert hands.

In some cases, you're required to soak in the natural surroundings or in particular plants prior to the ceremony in order to make sure you're clean before beginning. If you go to the Amazon in the Amazon, you'll almost definitely be in the open under an open-sided house that has only a roof, referred to as a maloka, so it is easy to connect with the natural world.

Other shamans consider performing cleansing and purging of the body prior to when the ceremony starts by making use of sacred tobacco leaves, known as mapacho, which induces the purging effects. Once you are to the event, you're capable of focusing in the process rather than being a victim of the purge for throughout the duration. The act of cleansing prior to the ceremony reduces the quantity of purging that happens during the drinking of ayahuasca tea.

It is highly recommended that you be in a calm mental state prior to beginning the ceremony. It is recommended to concentrate on breathing, or do meditation in order to calm and clear your mind. The ceremonies focus on healing, spiritual and focused. It helps you stay in a positive space within your mind and heart prior to taking part in the ceremony.

As the ceremony gets underway the ceremony, it may take a moment for everyone to discuss their goals. The Shaman is then able to bless the tea prior to serving it each person at the time of ceremony. The Shaman will invoke protection from negativity and provides an avenue for spirits to utilize the tea to heal energy by blowing sacred smoke of the mapacho to the tea. Additionally, he will use Agua Florida, or Palo Santo incense to consecrate the tea. After that, he will invite everyone to join in an order to begin the process of dispensing the drink.

In all likelihood this brew is described as having an extremely bitter and earthy flavor and isn't something to enjoy if consumed. You should swiftly take a sip and make careful not to be vomiting for at least 15 minutes to ensure that the drink can fully get into your system.

It is likely that if you take more than one drink that the initial dose is lower to allow your body to become used to the medication and to build an association to the grapevine. It is to also ensure that your experience does not get you into an intense sensory state making it difficult to handle certain scenarios in your initial session. The best way to handle these situations is to go slow with these situations since they may take a while to absorb.

When everyone has drunk after which the Shaman will take a sip and makes the room dark, burning the candles being utilized. It is your choice to move about as you wish, but it is suggested that you lie down on mats that are made available so you can relax in this quiet place. There are usually other things to help you relax throughout the event, such as pillows and towels. Also, you may be offered the water infused with plants to maintain your levels of hydration.

This is the stage at which you begin feeling your effects from the drink can be described as mariacion. This is the time when you enter into the fourth dimension, which puts your in touch with various spirit beings of plants. The Shaman may invite as many as forty of the plant spirits who teach help in healing the time. They work with the Shaman to make sure the area is cleansed of any negative energy as well as to ensure the area is protected.

Their presence is essential to the ceremony because the spirit plants collaborate together with Madre Ayahuasca, who collaborates with the Shaman to open the way for the root of disease or trauma to manifest physically.

If about 30 minutes have passed and the benefits of Ayahuasca begin to become evident and the Shaman begins singing the icanos in order to transform your thoughts into a state that will improve the visions Mother Ayahuasca will provide you with.

The songs and chants are unique to master plants since they are called upon to enter into the sacred area that is the part of the ceremony, to assist in the development of connections and visions you get. The icano is also a symbol to honor Mother Ayahuasca who is brought into the ceremony to serve as the guru of all other spirit plants in the ceremony. The only thing that could happen is singing chants which the shaman sings, or facilitators could include a mouth harp, drums or even maracas to the area.

As soon as the music kicks in at this point, you will begin to feel the drug begin to move across your body as snakes. The feeling will be an intense tug-of-war between fever and cold and it is possible to experience the burning sensation of negative thoughts begin to creep up.

In order to purge it is common to have smaller pots at your area and tissues to use the bathroom or to clean your mouth. The experience isn't always the most pleasant scenario, however the relief is worth the effort once it's done because your mind will be more calm and clear. Mother Ayahuasca will be able to perform her best.

While you're there you begin to slip to a place that is extremely dreamy, yet grounded on the real life. It could seem like an end of life review due to the number of thoughts and pictures that pop up in your head. People can even lie on their backs and feel a trance between sleep and waking that's intense and surreal.

When the medication begins working it will begin to lose your sense of time. Additionally, your body could transform into a variety of species or even observe them in other people. Keep in mind not to be afraid, and remain open regardless of the things you see.

The usual way Spirit is able to communicate with you is through the form of an Anaconda. There is a feeling that you're being snared at beginning as she is being absorbed within the body of yours. The first time you can begin to communicate fully with her in that moment. When she has merged into your life, that is when you get rid of all which makes you fearful about your situation, as you'll experience an enlightening and enlightening experience.

There are certain times in the ceremony At certain points during the ceremony, during the ceremony, Shaman can blow smoke from tobacco or Palo Santo incense, to change the sacred space and push the participants in different directions throughout the process. This technique is referred to by soplar, and could be achieved when he is in his seat or by stepping in to blow this out individually for every participant. There is the possibility of having either a facilitator or Shaman himself come over to your home to talk with you during the ceremony. Additionally, some shamans come to your individual to help you with the work of the master plant personally. Shamans Shamans take the tense energies from the individual by performing Chupar through sucking the energies out of the individual as well as the process of soplar.

In the span of 4 to 6 hours it is possible to drift into and out of this state, whether awake and alert or lying in a bed, appearing asleep. But, you are fully awake and absorbing all the data as if it were sponges. The medication helps you examine yourself and the activities that you've accomplished in a clear light. This will allow you to remove the ties that these experiences have in your life and move forward using this knowledge better for everyone.

While all ceremonies vary according to the location of your ceremony and the beliefs of the Shaman conducting them, they generally take between 2 and four days. The ceremony itself can range between 3 and seven hours long.

The Shaman could begin to dance while singing icaros, while the entire group is seated in a circle in front of a bonfire. The burning of the fire serves as a purifying part and also a means to allow the Shaman to watch each participant throughout the ceremony and determine whether he should alter the tone by using new icaros or sacred incense or requires special attention.

There are different rules during the ceremony, based of the Shaman. The Shaman may invite participants to sing with him or require you to remain at a distance so that you can fully enjoy the moment. These are the rules of conduct that are understood prior to when the ceremony gets underway. If you aren't sure, make certain to inquire about you need to know about the specific ceremony you are planning.

As the Shaman sings and chanting, he's conversing with Spirits of The Master Plants to help heal and guide the attendees on a deeper scale. The Shaman is working together with all the master plant spirits because they work together along with The Spirit of Aya to fulfill the most powerful intention of all who participate in the ritual. If you've got a well skilled Shaman is competent to complete all of these tasks at once as they keep in the loop of each person's vitality.

If the Shaman is aware that you require special attention, but he isn't in a position to stop the many projects he's completing then he'll have his assistants assist him.

The rituals are held in the evening because the spirit animals are sleeping and it will allow you to connect through your Spirit of the Vine in a more clear way.

Then, after the ceremony following the ceremony, the Shaman is likely to conduct a cleansing ritual for every person who was part of the ceremony. The intention is to cleanse the body of any negative energy found in their subliminal energy body. The energies that are drawn to them due to the condition of vulnerability they're in.

The most popular choice is to be dressed in white at the time of wedding ceremonies.

www.ingramcontent.com/pod-product-compliance
Lightning Source LLC
Chambersburg PA
CBHW071332120626
46546CB00002B/533